New Insights into Systemic Sclerosis

Edited by Michal Tomcik

Published in London, United Kingdom

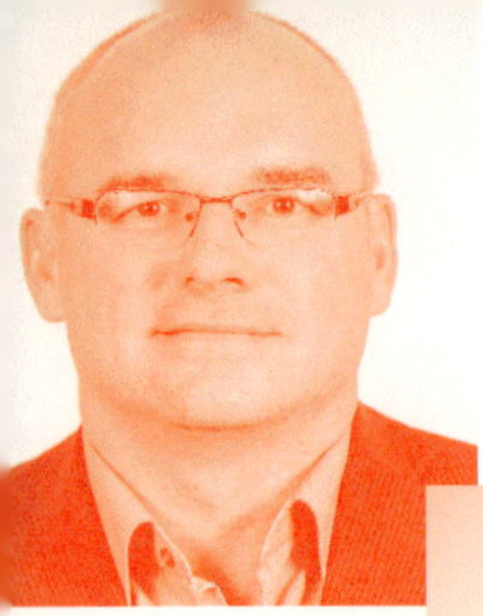
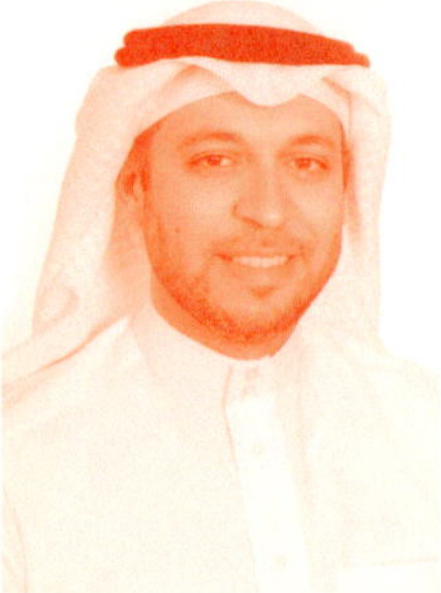
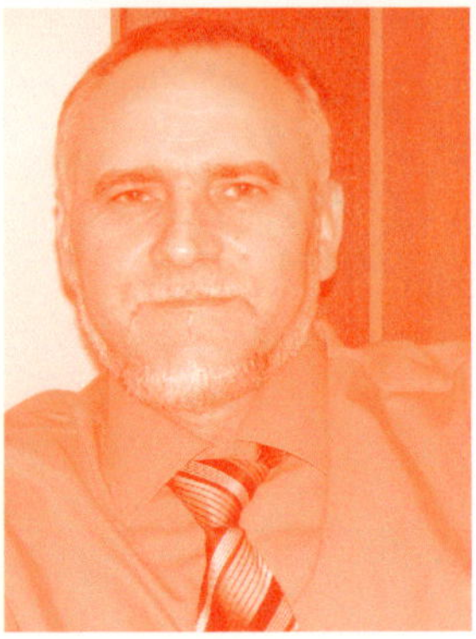
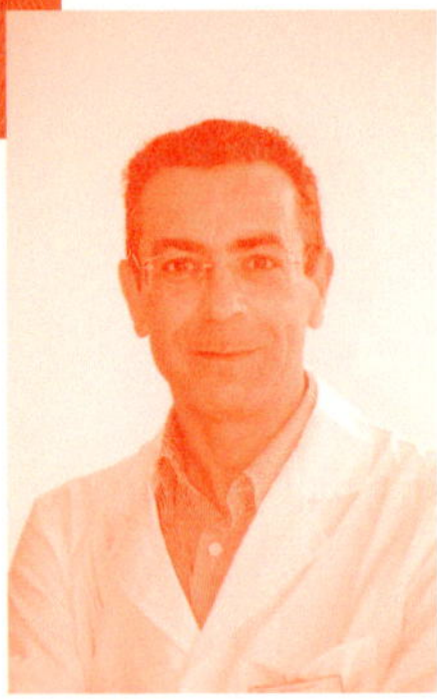
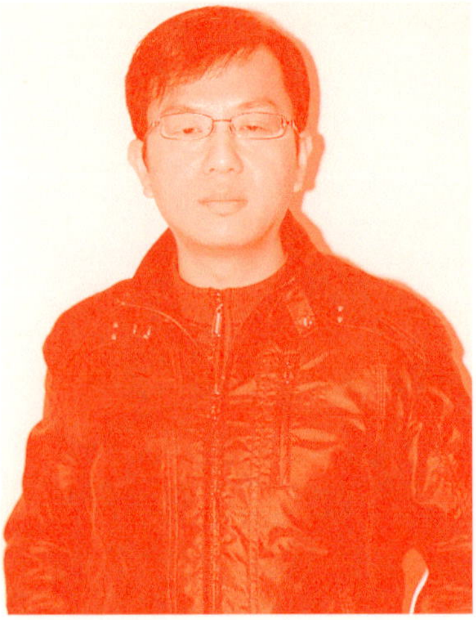
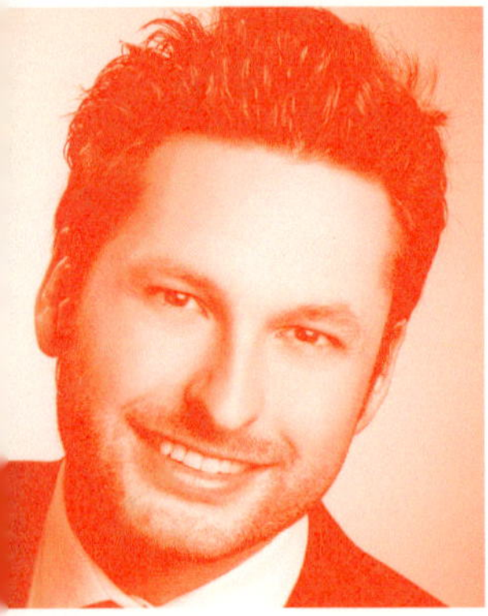
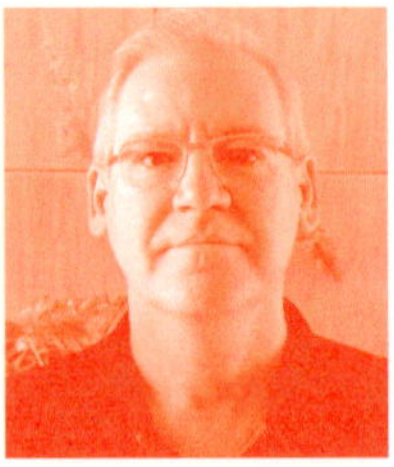

IntechOpen

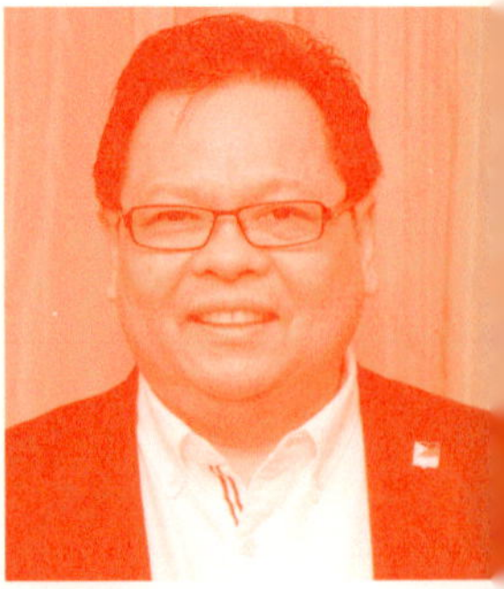
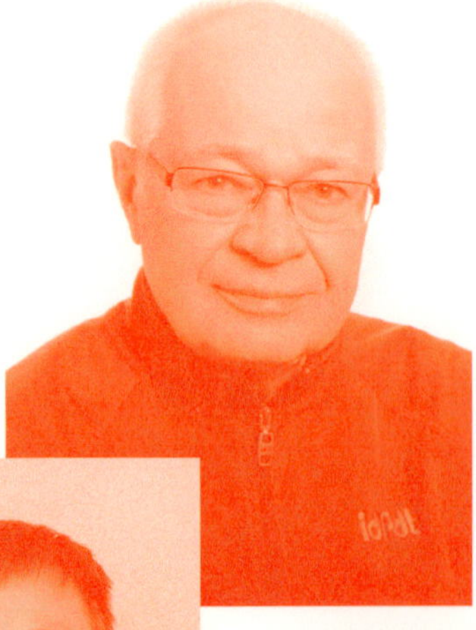
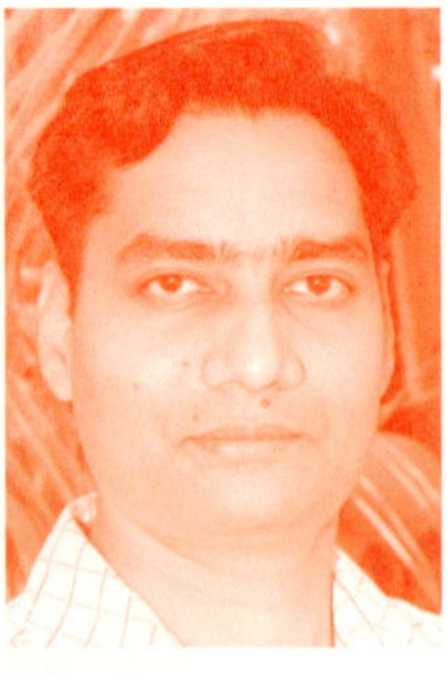
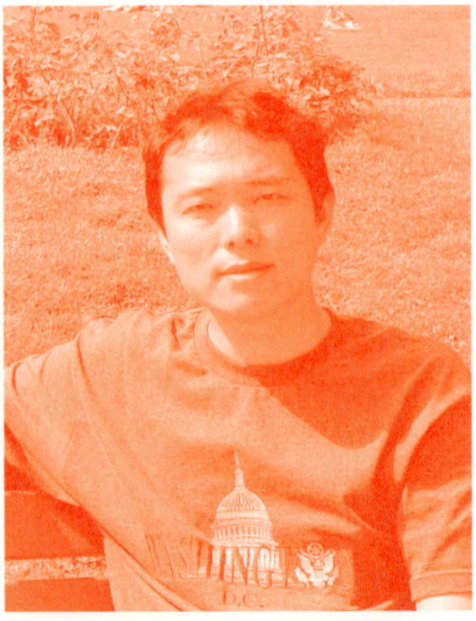
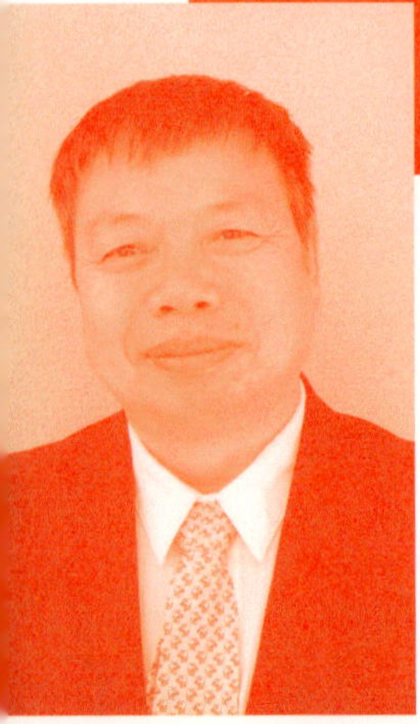
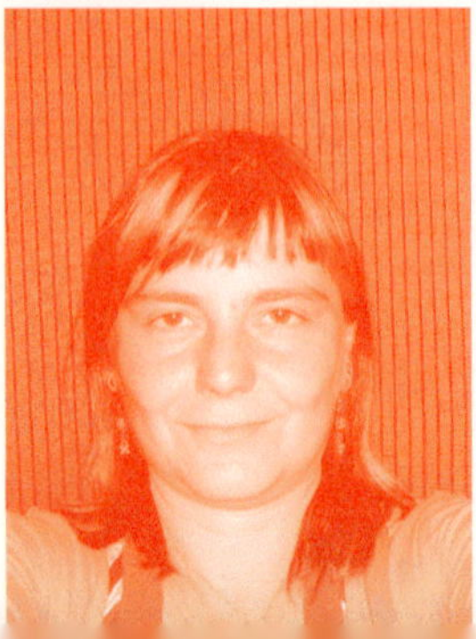

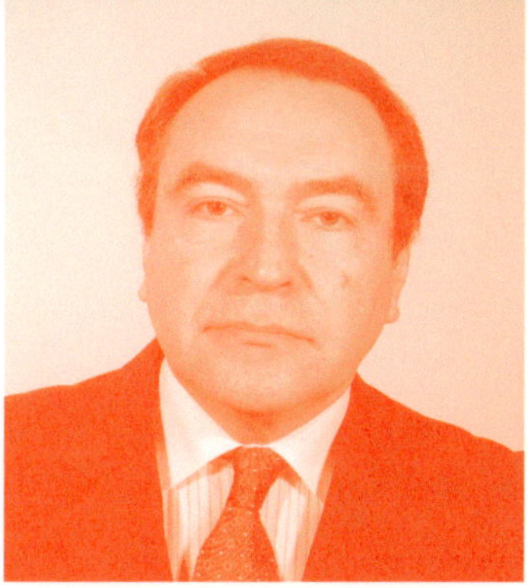
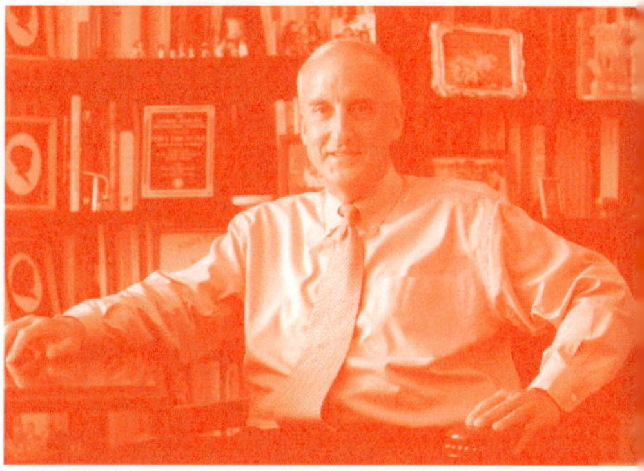
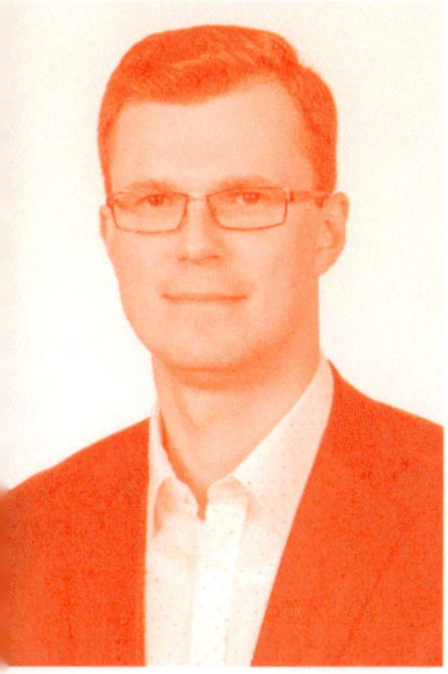
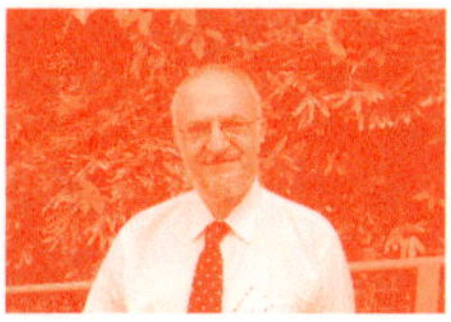
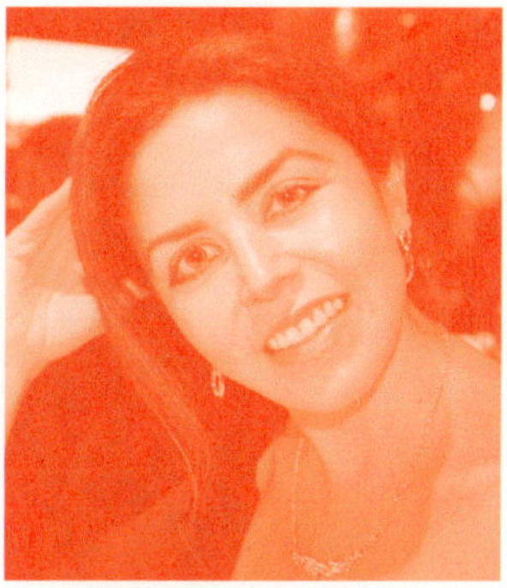

Supporting open minds since 2005

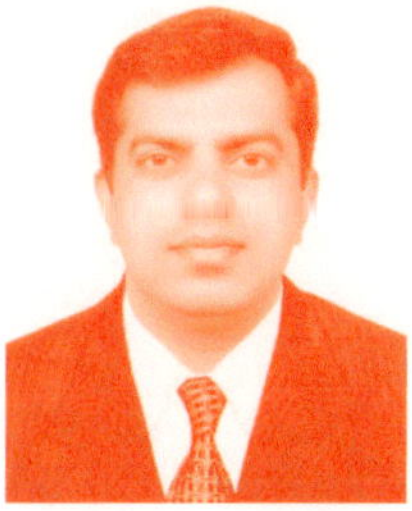
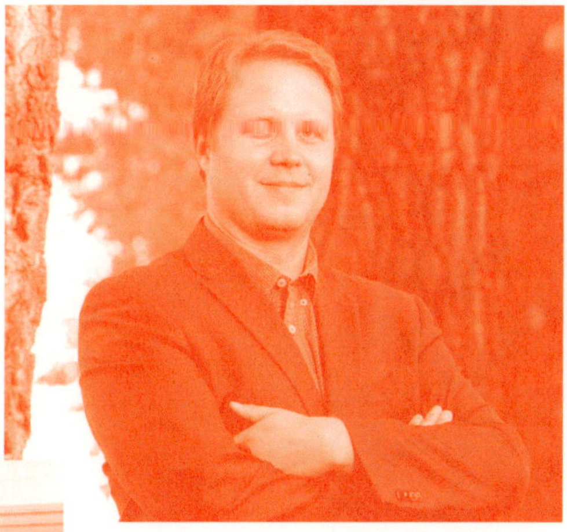
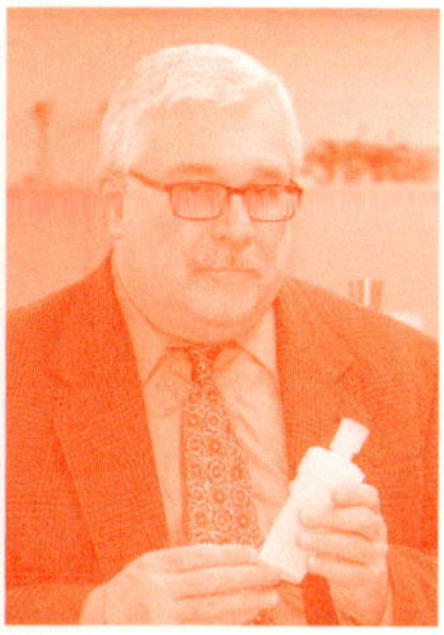
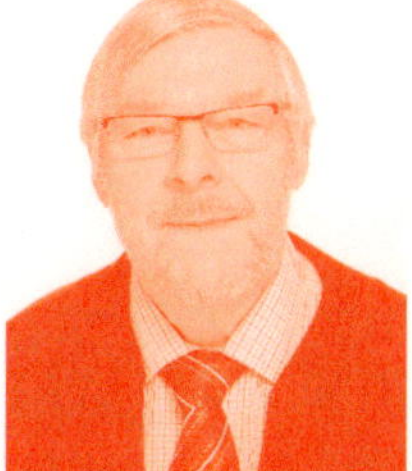
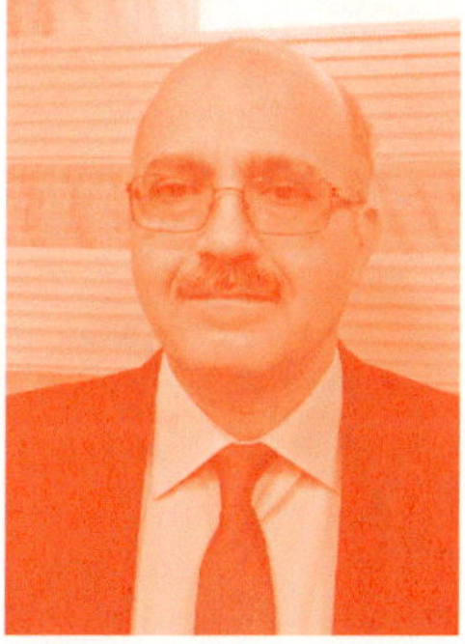
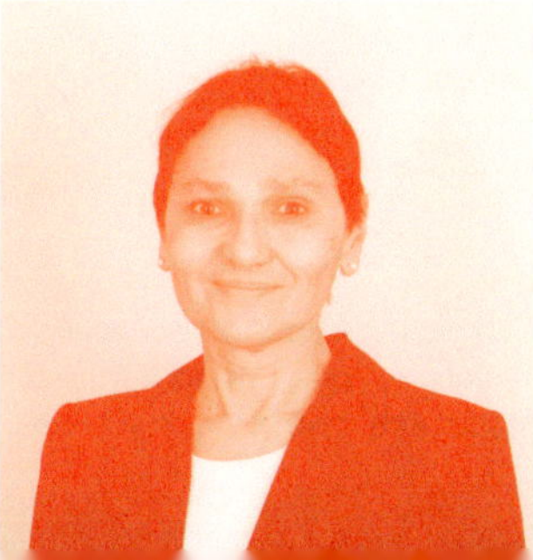
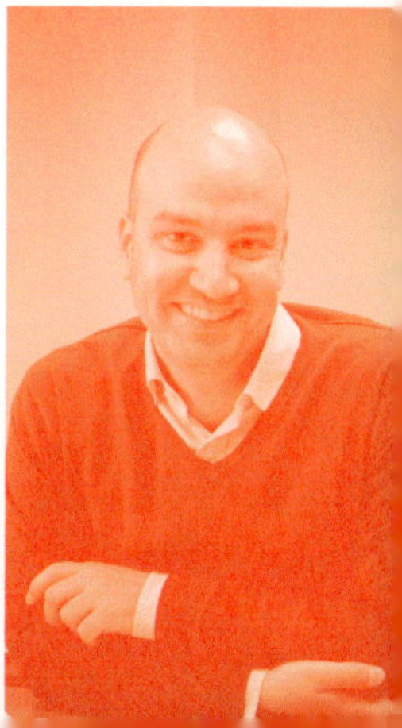

New Insights into Systemic Sclerosis
http://dx.doi.org/10.5772/intechopen.78254
Edited by Michal Tomcik

Contributors
John Swisher, Shashank Kailash, Maja Špiritović, Sabina Oreska, Michal Tomcik, Barbora Hermankova, Tomas Soukup, Jan Tomš, Roman Šafránek, Ondrej Kodet

First published in London, United Kingdom, 2019 by IntechOpen
IntechOpen is the global imprint of INTECHOPEN LIMITED, registered in England and Wales, registration number: 11086078, The Shard, 25th floor, 32 London Bridge Street
London, SE19SG - United Kingdom
Printed in Croatia

British Library Cataloguing-in-Publication Data
A catalogue record for this book is available from the British Library

Additional hard and PDF copies can be obtained from orders@intechopen.com

New Insights into Systemic Sclerosis
Edited by Michal Tomcik
p. cm.
Print ISBN 978-1-83962-204-5
Online ISBN 978-1-83962-205-2
eBook (PDF) ISBN 978-1-83962-206-9

For EU product safety concerns:
IN TECH d.o.o., Prolaz Marije Krucifikse Kozulić 3, 51000 Rijeka, Croatia, info@intechopen.com or visit our website at intechopen.com.

Meet the editor

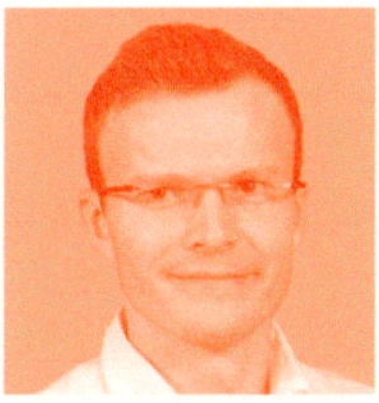

Associate Professor Michal Tomčík, MD, PhD, is a young board-certified rheumatologist working at the Institute of Rheumatology in Prague, teaching pregraduate students and supervising postgraduate students at the Department of Rheumatology, First Faculty of Medicine, Charles University, Prague, Czech Republic. His PhD and associate professor theses were focused on novel targets of antifibrotic therapy in systemic sclerosis. He is a member of the Czech Society for Rheumatology and EUSTAR. He is the author/coauthor of over 65 publications, 15 book chapters, and two books. His interests in clinical and basic research comprise systemic sclerosis, idiopathic inflammatory myopathies, rheumatoid arthritis, spondyloarthropathies, novel targets of antifibrotic therapy, biomarkers, non-pharmacological interventions, atherosclerosis and cardiovascular risk, body composition, and sexual dysfunctions.

Contents

Preface

Systemic sclerosis (scleroderma) is the most enigmatic and challenging of all rheumatic diseases. To date, it is considered incurable and carries the highest cause-specific mortality of all the connective tissue diseases. Despite the advancements in basic, translational, and clinical research that have been made in recent years, the etiology and pathophysiology of this complex and heterogeneous condition remain to be elucidated. The pathogenesis of scleroderma involves an interplay between genetic, epigenetic, and environmental factors that cause alterations in the immune and vascular systems and lead to progressive tissue fibrosis. The heterogeneity, highly variable clinical presentations, multisystemic manifestations, natural history, response to treatment, low prevalence, and level of public awareness or government investment represent some of the reasons for slow progress in the field of systemic sclerosis. Despite the large numbers of clinical trials and the progress made in their design over the last decade, no approved disease-modifying therapies exist for scleroderma to date. Currently available pharmacological therapies predominantly target inflammatory and vascular pathways, have variable and unpredictable clinical efficacy, usually undesirable safety profiles, and only a modest effect on long-term survival. All of these factors contribute to the significant impact of this challenging disease on the quality of life of patients with scleroderma and their families. Nevertheless, life expectancy of scleroderma patients has improved over recent years, mainly because of better disease management and efficacy of available treatment modalities for organ manifestations and complications. However, there is a large unmet need for increasing the awareness of systemic sclerosis among patients, physicians, and allied health professionals, and for comprehensive multidisciplinary care, which should include physical and occupational therapy, and optimization of nutrition, sleep, and sexual or psychological aspects to reduce suffering and disability of scleroderma patients.

This book covers novel insights into the pathogenetic mechanisms, classification, differential diagnosis, diagnostic methods, clinical management, and available treatment approaches of a number of major organ manifestations of scleroderma, including pulmonary hypertension and gastrointestinal and renal involvement. Furthermore, it provides a comprehensive overview of often neglected aspects such as scleroderma-like syndromes, and the impact of sexual and biopsychosocial issues on the ability of patients to participate in society and to work. Contributors include well-established scleroderma experts, rheumatologists, internal medicine specialists, a pathologist and dermatologist, young research fellows, and experienced physiotherapists with an interest in basic, translational, and clinical research in systemic sclerosis. I am indebted to my colleagues for their dedication, expertise, and timely submissions and believe that their contributions reflect the progress made over the last couple of years in understanding and managing systemic sclerosis.

I would like to express my gratitude to all colleagues, research collaborators, my students and mentors in rheumatology, and to all the patients who have taught me about scleroderma and were sources of inspiration over the years.

I gratefully acknowledge Ana Pantar for the kind invitation to become an academic editor of this book and the Author Service Manager Edi Lipović for his dedicated technical assistance, patience, readiness, and helpfulness.

I am deeply grateful and indebted to my family for their ongoing support, encouragement, patience, and love.

New Insights into Systemic Sclerosis aims to provide students, residents, trainees, researchers, rheumatologists, and other specialists interested in this fascinating disease with up-to-date knowledge and concepts spanning pathogenesis to the clinical management of scleroderma.

Michal Tomčík, MD, PhD
Associate Professor at the Department of Rheumatology,
First Faculty of Medicine, Charles University,
Institute of Rheumatology,
Prague, Czech Republic

Chapter 1

Advances in Management of Pulmonary Hypertension Associated with Systemic Sclerosis

John W. Swisher and Shashank Kailash

Abstract

Pulmonary hypertension is a well-known complication of systemic sclerosis. Patients with systemic sclerosis may develop a pulmonary arteriopathy characterized by vascular remodeling, increased pulmonary vascular resistance, and right ventricular failure. Pulmonary hypertension may also arise in systemic sclerosis as a consequence of interstitial lung disease or left ventricular dysfunction. Vascular remodeling is more prevalent than other forms of pulmonary hypertension in systemic sclerosis. The pathogenesis of pulmonary vascular remodeling in this disease state is not completely understood; however, there is evidence of a complex process involving genetic susceptibility, risk factors, vascular injury, and endothelial dysfunction. In those patients with pulmonary arterial hypertension, survival prognosis is extremely poor if the diagnosis is delayed or goes undetected and untreated. In recent years, a number of disease-targeted therapies have been developed that improve functional capacity, hemodynamics, and survival. Early detection and treatment with one or more targeted therapies are essential to improving survival when systemic sclerosis is complicated by pulmonary arterial hypertension.

Keywords: pulmonary arterial hypertension, systemic sclerosis, endothelin, nitric oxide, prostacyclin

1. Introduction

Systemic sclerosis (SSc) is a multisystem, autoimmune disease characterized by excessive collagen deposition and fibrosis of the skin and internal organs. The autoimmune process may affect the lungs with the development of interstitial fibrosis, pulmonary hypertension, or both. Pulmonary hypertension (PH) may result from a pathologic process of remodeling in the pulmonary arteries, in which case it is referred to as pulmonary arterial hypertension (PAH). Pulmonary hypertension may also arise secondary to interstitial fibrosis with chronic hypoxemia or myocardial fibrosis with postcapillary pulmonary hypertension. Pulmonary arterial hypertension associated with systemic sclerosis (SSc-PAH) represents the second most common cause of PAH after the idiopathic form of the disease (iPAH). Pulmonary arterial hypertension is associated with a progressive rise in pulmonary vascular resistance that can result in right ventricular failure and death. Patients with SSc-PAH have higher mortality than the idiopathic form of PAH or PAH associated with other diseases, such as congenital heart disease. While there is a reasonable amount of information available pertaining to SSc-PAH, much of what we know about PAH in general comes from investigations of the idiopathic form of the disease. The current chapter will review current knowledge about PAH in the patient with systemic sclerosis and contrast it with information that distinguishes SSc-PAH from the idiopathic form of PAH.

2. Epidemiology

The prevalence of systemic sclerosis-associated PAH is reported to be between 5 and 15% of patients with systemic sclerosis [1–3]. There is wide variability in reported prevalence rates which range from as low as 3.7% [4] to as high as 43% [5]. This variability is in large part due to methods used to establish the diagnosis of pulmonary hypertension. While some prevalence studies base reported findings on echocardiography, others confirm diagnosis with right heart catheterization. Right heart catheterization (RHC) is the gold standard for accurate diagnosis of pulmonary hypertension and for distinguishing pulmonary arterial from postcapillary hypertension. Prevalence rates are consistently lower when diagnosis is determined by right heart catheterization [6]. In a meta-analysis, Yang et al. found 12 studies reporting the prevalence of PAH in SSc ranging from 3.6 to 32% with a pooled prevalence of 13%. Five of the 12 studies confirmed the diagnosis of PAH with right heart catheterization yielding a pooled prevalence estimate of 8.2%, while the pooled prevalence estimate from seven studies relying on echocardiography was 18% [7]. Even when pulmonary hypertension is diagnosed by right heart catheterization, some patients in cohort studies may refuse to undergo catheterization, thus affecting true prevalence [8].

The prevalence of pulmonary hypertension in systemic sclerosis depends on the phenotypic form of systemic sclerosis and the pathophysiologic mechanism behind the development of PH. The Australian Scleroderma Cohort Study (ASCS) of 232 patients identified PH in 10.1% of patients with diffuse scleroderma and in 12.7% of those with the limited form of the disease [9]. Prevalence of SSc-PAH consistently exceeds interstitial lung disease-PH (ILD-PH) or postcapillary-PH (PC-PH). Evaluation of PH subtypes in the ASCS cohort revealed 83.6% with PAH, 2.2% with ILD-PH, and 7.8% with PC-PH. The DETECT study, which was designed to develop an algorithm for detection of PAH in SSc, included 145 patients all of whom underwent right heart catheterization revealing 19% with PAH, 6% with ILD-PH, and 6% with PC-PH [10]. An Italian cohort of 867 consecutive SSc patients included 69 patients confirmed to have pulmonary hypertension with point prevalence for PAH 3.7%, PH secondary to ILD 1.4%, and postcapillary-PH 1.3% [4]. The lower prevalence of PH in the Italian cohort study raised speculation that ethnic factors might influence the prevalence of PH in SSc.

Prevalence of SSc-PAH appears to depend on other factors, such as duration of systemic sclerosis, gender, and ethnicity. Observations in the Pulmonary Hypertension Assessment and Recognition of Outcomes in Scleroderma (PHAROS) study suggested patients who were female, Caucasian, or suffering with limited cutaneous scleroderma were more likely to have PAH [11]. Additionally, a reduction in DLCO below 55% predicted was noted in 79% of patients with SSc-PAH compared to 55% of patients with SSc alone. Other authors have observed a greater chance of developing SSc-PAH in male patients age 47 or older [12], patients with SSC more than 10 years [13], and those with DLCO <55% [14]. Iudici suggested that systemic sclerosis patients of Italian descent may be less likely to develop pulmonary hypertension based on observations that prevalence rates were substantially lower than those reported in Anglo-Saxon patients [4].

3. Pathophysiology

3.1 WHO classification of pulmonary hypertensive diseases

The World Health Organization (WHO) has classified pulmonary hypertension into five distinct groups on the basis of the primary pathophysiologic mechanism leading to elevated pulmonary artery pressure (**Table 1**) [15]. In a generic sense, pulmonary hypertension is diagnosed when mean pulmonary artery pressure (mPAP) ≥ 25 mmHg is measured by pulmonary artery catheterization. Patients classified as WHO Group 1 develop an arteriopathy of the small precapillary pulmonary arteries characterized by endothelial proliferation, smooth muscle layer hypertrophy, in situ thrombosis, and formation of plexiform lesions (**Figure 1**). Pulmonary arterial hypertension is defined more specifically as a mPAP ≥25 mmHg and also a capillary wedge pressure (CWP) ≤ 15 mmHg and pulmonary vascular resistance (PVR) > 3 Wood units (WU) [16]. Those in WHO Group 2 have elevated pulmonary artery pressure with a postcapillary origin typically related to left heart disease or dysfunction. WHO Group 3 pulmonary hypertension is a consequence of chronic hypoxia and attendant vasoconstriction as seen in chronic lung diseases, such as pulmonary fibrosis or emphysema. The fourth WHO Group constitutes those with pulmonary vascular obstruction, most often due to chronic thromboembolic disease. Finally, WHO Group 5 is a group of patients with pulmonary hypertension of mixed etiologies that do not fit within the other categories.

3.2 Histopathology

Patients who develop the characteristic vasculopathy of WHO Group 1 PAH experience a progressive rise in pulmonary vascular resistance resulting from the gradual occlusion of smaller vessels by cellular hyperproliferation, thrombosis, and plexiform lesion formation that obstruct blood flow. The resulting rise in resistance to blood flow through the pulmonary circulation causes right ventricular strain with initial compensation and hypertrophy. Eventually the rising resistance overwhelms the right ventricle resulting in its failure.

Pulmonary hypertension as it occurs in the scleroderma spectrum of diseases can develop by virtue of one or more mechanisms and can be classified as WHO Group 1 with the characteristic features of a precapillary arteriopathy, as WHO Group 2 when scleroderma affects myocardial physiology, or as WHO Group 3 if the patient primarily suffers from interstitial fibrosis and hypoxemia. Patients with systemic sclerosis may have complex forms of pulmonary hypertension involving more than one of these mechanisms. Treatment is dependent on the mechanism or mechanisms behind rising pulmonary vascular resistance, so it is important to carefully establish the root cause, or causes, for pulmonary hypertension in this patient population. Pulmonary arterial hypertension is the most common form of pulmonary hypertension to affect patients with systemic sclerosis. Therefore, this chapter's focus is primarily on the pathogenesis of pulmonary arterial hypertension. While other mechanisms leading to pulmonary hypertension in this group will be reviewed, the development of SSc-PAH is a devastating complication, and the greatest body of information available pertains to the WHO Group 1 type of arteriopathy.

Characteristic histopathologic features of pulmonary vascular remodeling observed in the patient with WHO Group 1 PAH are well-described and involve all layers of the pulmonary arterial vessels (**Figure 1A**) [17, 19, 21]. It is not uncommon for a similar process to affect the postcapillary venules in systemic sclerosis. A majority of patients will have in situ vessel thrombosis [18]. Flow-limiting

1.	**Pulmonary Arterial Hypertension**		
	1.1	Idiopathic	
	1.2	Heritable	
		1.2.1	BMPR2 mutation
		1.2.2	Other mutations
	1.3	Drug and toxin induced	
	1.4	Associated with:	
		1.4.1	Connective tissue disease
		1.4.2	Human immunodeficiency virus (HIV) infection
		1.4.3	Portal hypertension
		1.4.4	Congenital heart disease
		1.4.5	Schistosomiasis
1′.	**Pulmonary veno-occlusive disease and/or pulmonary capillary hemangiomatosis**		
	1′.1	Idiopathic	
	1′.2	Heritable	
		1′.2.1	EIF2AK4 mutation
		1′.2.2	Other mutations
	1′.3	Drugs, toxins and radiation induced	
	1′.4	Assoicated with:	
		1′.4.1	Connective tissue disease
		1′.4.2	HIV infection
1″.	**Persistant pulmonary hypertension of the newborn**		
2.	**Pulmonary Hypertension Due to Left Heart Disease**		
	2.1	Left ventricular systolic dysfunction	
	2.2	Left ventricular diastolic dysfunction	
	2.3	Valvular heart disease	
	2.4	Congenital/acquired left heart inflow/outflow tract obstruction and Congenital cardiomyopathies	
	2.5	Congenital/acquired pulmonary vein stenosis	
3.	**Pulmonary Hypertension Due to Lung Diseases and/or Hypoxia**		
	3.1	Chronic obstructive pulmonary disease	
	3.2	Interstitial lung disease	
	3.3	Other pulmonary diseases with mixed obstructive and restrictive components	
	3.4	Sleep-disordered breathing	
	3.5	Alveolar hypoventilation	
	3.6	Chronic high altitude exposure	
	3.7	Developmental lung diseases	
4.	**Chronic Thromboembolic Pulmonary Hypertension and Other Pulmonary Artery Obstructions**		
	4.1	Chronic thromboembolic pulmonary hypertension	
	4.2	Other pulmonary artery obstructions	
		4.2.1	Angiosarcoma
		4.2.2	Other intravascualar tumors
		4.2.3	Arteritis
		4.2.4	Congenital pulmonary arteries stenoses
		4.2.5	Parasites
5.	**Pulmonary Hypertension With Unclear and/or Multifactorial Mechanisms**		
	5.1	Hematologic disorders: chronic hemolytic anemia, myeloproliferative disorders, splenectomy	
	5.2	Systemic disorders: sarcoidosis, pulmonary histiocytosis, lymphangioleiomyomatosis	
	5.3	Metabolic disorders: glycogen storage disease, Gaucher disease, thyroid disorders	
	5.4	Other: pulmonary tumoral thrombotic microangiopathy, fibrosing mediastinitis, chronic renal failure	

Table 1.
The World Health Organization classification of pulmonary hypertensive diseases.

pathologic features involving the intimal layer of the pulmonary arteries include eccentric or concentric intimal thickening and formation of plexiform or angiomatoid lesions (**Figure 1B**) [17, 19, 21]. There is excessive cell proliferation and

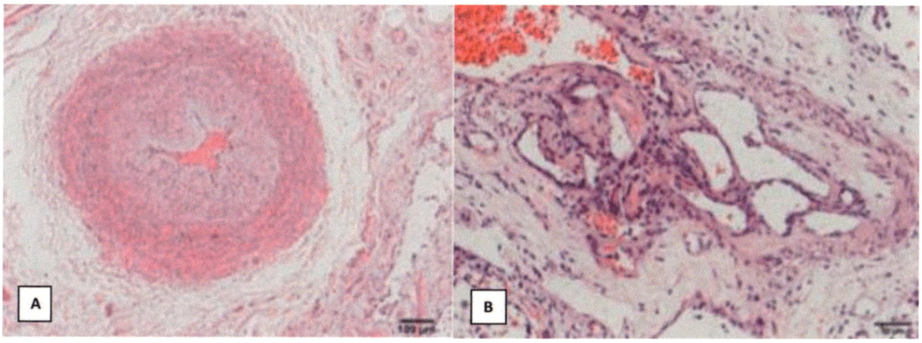

Figure 1.
Histopathology of vascular remodeling in pulmonary arterial hypertension. (A) Medial hypertrophy and cellular intimal thickening. (B) Fibrin thrombi in glomoid plexiform lesion. Reprinted by permission from Springer Nature: Ishibashi-Ueda and Ohta-Ogo [21]. Copyright 2017.

hypertrophy of the smooth muscle layer. Thickening of the adventitial layer, primarily due to collagen deposition, is also noted in these patients [17, 19–21].

Areas of eccentric intimal thickening may represent fibrotic organization of localized thrombi. This concept is supported by observations of myofibroblast infiltration and accumulation of mucopolysaccharides in these localized lesions along the vessel lumen [17]. Eccentric intimal lesions of this nature have been demonstrated in lung explants from patients with severe idiopathic PAH and those with the CREST (calcinosis, Raynaud phenomenon, esophageal dysmotility, sclerodactyly, and telangiectasias) variant of scleroderma [22]. Vascular resistance is also increased by concentric proliferation of the endothelial cell layer creating the well-described "onion skin" lesion that is thought to involve myofibroblasts and smooth muscle cells (SMC), as well as endothelial cells [23, 24]. Plexiform lesions consist of complex vascular networks with a myofibroblast core which distorts the vessel wall as it expands and extends into the lumen and the connective tissues surrounding the vessel [23]. A rosary of dilated channels may form an angiomatoid, or dilation, lesion and obstruct arterial flow [25]. Although specific mechanisms involved in intimal remodeling are yet to be defined with clarity, it is largely believed that the processes begin with endothelial injury and, in genetically susceptible individuals, result in endothelial proliferation, smooth muscle cell and myofibroblast migration, decreased apoptosis, and deposition of extracellular matrix [17, 18, 26].

Normally, the medial layer of muscularized arteries accounts for about 10–15% of the outer arterial diameter, while in iPAH, it may be 30–60% of the outside diameter [20, 27]. Thickening of the medial layer is largely due to cell hypertrophy; however, hyperplasia of the smooth muscle cells and accumulation of extracellular matrix also contribute to the shift in tunica media dimension [17, 28]. Non-muscularized arteries may become muscularized with peripheral extension of proximal smooth muscle cell segments and pericyte differentiation into smooth muscle cells [19].

The adventitial layer is comprised of fibroblasts and extracellular matrix (ECM) components. While it accounts for roughly 15% of vessel diameter under normal circumstances, it may represent double that in the patient with PAH [17]. In addition to its role in providing structural support for the vessel, there is evidence that inflammatory cells and extracellular matrix components of the adventitia may serve a role in the regulation of cell activities in other layers [29]. Typical components of the pulmonary vascular ECM include elastin, collagens, fibronectin, tenascin, thrombospondin, growth factors, and matrix metalloproteinases and proteoglycans [30]. Normal vessel structural and functional integrity depend on a balance between ECM deposition and degradation. Turnover is regulated by matrix metalloproteinases, adamalysins, serine elastase, and endogenous enzyme inhibitors [31]. In PAH excessive deposition of ECM contributes to vascular remodeling and decreased vessel wall compliance. Examination of the pulmonary vascular ECM in iPAH reveals prominent deposition of collagens I and III, enhanced collagen metabolism, alterations in proteoglycans and elastin, upregulation of tenascin C which is involved in intimal hyperplasia, and modification of fibronectin contributing to SMC proliferation and migration [32–35]. Scleroderma is a disease characterized by overproduction of ECM, although there have been no studies detailing ECM composition in SSc-PAH.

Studies comparing the pathologic features of iPAH to those with connective tissue disease- associated PAH (CTD-PAH), and specifically SSc-PAH, have highlighted both similarities and differences between the groups. In a study of lung explants from transplant recipients, Stacher et al. compared the features of vascular remodeling in patients with iPAH and CTD-PAH [36]. The investigators noted more pronounced morphologic changes in the smaller-sized and precapillary arteries in CTD-PAH. Plexiform lesions were noted with similar frequency but had a more scattered distribution in the patients with connective tissue disease. Histopathologic studies comparing these patient groups also reveal more active interstitial inflammation and fibrosis in systemic sclerosis and other connective tissue diseases [19, 36, 37]. In a study comparing tissue from 24 patients with SSc-PAH and 9 iPAH patients, Argula et al. noted fewer plexiform lesions and more interstitial cellularity and fibrosis in the SSc-PAH group, while there was little difference in intimal proliferation or arteriolar smooth muscle hypertrophy [37]. In contrast, Overbeek and colleagues found no plexiform lesions in a group of patients with limited cutaneous systemic sclerosis and PAH, while these lesions were present in 10 of 11 comparative iPAH patients [38]. Further intimal fibrosis and fibrosis of the pulmonary veins and venules were observed with significantly higher frequency in SSc-PAH. While there are similarities in the overall pattern of vascular remodeling in iPAH and SSc-PAH, differences are notable and suggest distinct pathogenetic mechanisms may be in play. Additionally, inflammation and fibrosis may have a greater role in SSc-PAH.

3.3 Pathogenesis

The coordinated mechanisms leading to vascular remodeling in PAH have been the subject of intensive investigation in recent years. It has been 18 years since Gaine proposed a theoretical model of the pathogenesis of PAH [18]. This model continues to serve as a basis for our basic understanding of the pathobiology of the disease and has been a platform for the development of approved therapies for WHO Group 1 PAH in use today. The model suggests a convergence of factors including genetic susceptibility, exposure to risk factors, vascular injury, and endothelial dysfunction leading to progressive remodeling of vasculature and rising pulmonary vascular resistance.

3.3.1 Genetic mutations

Evidence of a genetic basis for PAH was first reported in 2000 with the discovery of the bone morphogenetic protein receptor II (*BMPR2*) gene mutation in patients with heritable PAH [39, 40]. Mutation of this gene has been identified in at least 70–80% of cases of heritable PAH and 15–25% of sporadic iPAH [41]. *BMPR2* protein concentrations are decreased by 75% in lung tissue and endothelial cells from subjects with PAH [24]. Other gene mutations related to *BMPR2* and its downstream signaling pathway are now known including mutations in *ALK1*, *ENG*, and genes encoding components of the SMAD downstream signaling pathway [19, 41].

Mutations unrelated to the *BMPR2* signaling pathway have also been identified in a very small percentage of PAH patients and include *KCNK3*, which encodes a pH-sensitive potassium channel, and *CAV1*, which encodes a membrane protein, caveolin 1, which is essential for the formation of lipid rafts or caveolae [41]. While no link between the development of SSc-PAH and mutation of *BMPR2* has been established, other unique mutations have been identified in the systemic sclerosis population with PAH. For instance, a rare functional polymorphism in the *TLR2* gene, which promotes induction of interleukin-6 (IL-6) and tumor necrosis factor-alpha (TNF-alpha), is associated with the development of PAH in systemic sclerosis [42]. The development of diffuse cutaneous scleroderma, fibrosing alveolitis, and PAH has been linked to polymorphisms in *TNFAIP3*, which regulates the NF-kB inflammatory pathway [43]. Genetic variation in the promoter region of *UPAR*, the urokinase-type plasminogen activator receptor, has been associated with digital ulceration and PAH in scleroderma patients [44]. Clearly, there is evidence for genetic susceptibility to develop PAH in systemic sclerosis, although genetic mechanisms appear to differ from those associated with iPAH.

BMPR2 is a member of the transforming growth factor-beta (TGF-beta) superfamily of genes and normally functions to limit proliferation of smooth muscle cells and enhance endothelial cell survival by inhibiting apoptosis [45]. In contrast, TGF-beta is thought to promote SMC proliferation, matrix deposition, and alterations in endothelial cell growth [46, 47]. TGF-beta is known for fibrotic effects in several disease states, among which are systemic sclerosis [48]. Evidence from investigations of heritable PAH and preclinical models of SSc suggests that endothelial injury and consequent pulmonary vasculopathy may arise from an imbalance in TGF-beta/BMP signaling pathways [49–53]. For example, reduced BMPR2 receptor expression in heritable PAH correlates with increased activity of TGF-beta and its downstream signaling pathways. Reduction in BMPR2 levels in patients with systemic sclerosis also correlates with enhanced activity of TGF-beta and downstream SMAD2 and MAPK signaling pathways. Based on these observations, a theory has been advanced that heightened TGF-beta activity in systemic sclerosis might suppress BMP signaling pathways that serve to protect the endothelium [19].

In addition to the disruption created by structural remodeling in the pulmonary vessels, endothelial injury and dysfunction may lead to imbalances in production of mediators that affect vascular tone and platelet aggregation and further regulate cell proliferation. Immunochemical studies have demonstrated reduced levels of nitric oxide synthase and prostacyclin synthase in the pulmonary vascular endothelium [54, 55]. These enzymes are critical to the endogenous production of nitric oxide and prostacyclin, both of which have vasodilatory and antiproliferative effects. The production of thromboxane is increased leading to enhanced vasoconstriction and in situ thrombosis [56]. Vasoconstriction and cell proliferation are promoted by increased production of endothelin-1 by pulmonary endothelium [57]. Endothelin-1, survivin, and vascular endothelial growth factor (VEGF) have been found in plexiform lesions and may augment endothelial and smooth muscle cell proliferation while limiting cell apoptosis [57–59]. Levels of nitric oxide synthase, prostacyclin synthase, and tumor suppressors, such as caveolin-1, are reduced in the plexiform lesions [54, 55, 60]. The imbalances in production of vasoactive mediators have largely driven the development of treatments designed to counteract these imbalances and improve pulmonary vascular resistance.

3.3.2 Serotonin

The role of serotonin in the pathogenesis of PAH has been a topic of interest and investigation for several years. Serotonin is thought to promote vasoconstriction and remodeling of pulmonary vessels by stimulating proliferation of SMCs and fibroblasts [61–63]. The induction of SMC proliferation may be affected by serotonin transporter activation of the platelet-derived growth factor-beta (PDGF-B) receptor [64]. In SSc patients, serotonin has been shown to induce ECM production by interstitial fibroblasts in a TGF-beta-dependent manner [65]. When a group of SSc-PAH patients were treated with ketanserin, a selective antagonist of S2 serotonergic receptors, a majority experienced reductions in pulmonary vascular resistance [66]. The serotonin pathway may hold promise for the development of new treatment approaches to SSc-PAH in the future.

3.3.3 Epigenetics

Epigenetic mechanisms affecting changes in cellular function in PAH have been a focus of more recent research. Epigenetic processes alter gene expression without effecting changes in DNA sequence. Epigenetic mechanisms may involve DNA methylation, modification of histone proteins, or RNA interference via microRNAs [67]. Extensive methylation of cytosine residues in the CpG dinucleotide sequences of the BMPR2 gene promoter region suppresses BMPR2 gene expression in SSc-PAH [68]. Elevated histone deacetylase levels have been noted in the lungs of PAH patients, and the inhibition of the deacetylase reduces proliferation of vascular fibroblasts and PDGF-stimulated SMC growth [69]. A number of microRNAs have been identified that influence cellular functions in hereditary and iPAH [19]. For instance, miR424 and miR503 normally suppress expression of fibroblast growth factor-2 (FGF-2); however, they are decreased in iPAH leading to an upregulation of FGF-2 expression [70]. These are just some representative examples of the growing knowledge of the role of epigenetic factors in PAH.

3.3.4 Cytokines and growth factors

The discovery of gene mutations involving the TGF-beta receptor family focused attention on the role of cytokines and growth factors in vascular remodeling of PAH. Observations of inflammatory cell infiltrates associated with vascular lesions and the presence of elevated cytokine levels in PAH have further supported a role for inflammation in this disease process. Lymphocytes, macrophages, dendritic cells, and mast cells have all been demonstrated on histopathologic examination of immune cell infiltrates in vascular lesions [17, 71, 72]. Elevated levels of several cytokines have been reported in iPAH including IL-1beta, IL-2, IL-4, IL-6, IL-8, IL-10, and IL-12p70, TNF-alpha, and chemokines CXC3L1, CCL2, and CCL5 [73–77]. The exact role of inflammation in the pathogenesis of PAH is unclear. Inflammation may reflect a consequence of hypoxia associated with PAH, as acute and chronic inflammation are known to occur in the setting of hypoxia. Alternatively, inflammatory mechanisms may be the drivers behind vascular cell injury and dysfunction. Macrophages are known to concentrate within and around advanced vascular lesions in iPAH and are thought to play a significant role in the remodeling process [78]. IL-6 produced by activated adventitial fibroblasts has been shown to induce a macrophage phenotype with proinflammatory and profibrotic characteristics [79]. Speculation about the role of immune dysregulation is supported by an observed deficiency of regulatory T cells in the lungs from iPAH patients [80]. In contrast to a deficiency of T-cell subpopulations, circulating autoantibodies and ectopic expansion of pulmonary lymphoid tissue in PAH patients suggest there is excessive B-cell activation [81]. PDGF has been implicated in the pathogenesis of PAH. Although originally discovered as a product of platelets, isoforms of this growth factor are also known to be secreted by macrophages, endothelial cells, SMCs, and fibroblasts [82]. PDGF is a potent mitogen and chemoattractant for endothelial cells, smooth muscle cells, and fibroblasts. PDGF receptor-beta expression is more intense in small and postcapillary vessels in SSc-PAH than iPAH [83]. The PDGF receptor antagonist, imatinib, was investigated for treatment of PAH, and during the initial study phase, improvements in hemodynamics and exercise capacity were noted. However, the long-term extension study was terminated early due to severe and unexpected adverse events including intracranial hemorrhage, death, and other side effects [84].

3.3.5 Autoantibodies

Autoantibodies against endothelial cell antigens may promote pulmonary vascular remodeling, especially in SSc-PAH. The expression of anti-endothelial cell antibodies and target antigens has been confirmed in iPAH and SSc-PAH, although the role of these antibodies in the pathogenesis of PAH remains undetermined [85, 86]. Anti-endothelial cell antibody levels in serum of connective tissue disease patients with or without PAH were evaluated by Li and colleagues compared with control subjects [87]. While endothelial cell antibodies were detected at similar levels in connective tissue disease patients irrespective of whether PAH was present, one specific endothelial antibody subtype (anti-22kD) was only found in the patients with PAH. A second subtype (anti-75kD) was noted at significantly higher levels in patients with PAH. The investigators concluded that these subtypes of endothelial antibody might indicate a more specific risk for PAH in connective tissue diseases. Tamby also demonstrated the presence of serum immunoglobulin anti-fibroblast antibodies in patients with iPAH and SSc-PAH with distinct reactivity against target antigens [88]. While these observations imply immunosuppressive therapy should be a treatment option for SSc-PAH and possibly iPAH, there is no evidence to date that this approach is beneficial. A prospective, multicenter trial to evaluate the effect of rituximab on disease progression in subjects with SSc-PAH receiving concurrent standard medical therapy is currently ongoing.

3.3.6 Cancer similarities

Certain features of pulmonary vascular cell dysfunction in patients with PAH have led to the suggestion that vascular remodeling may represent a cancer-like process involving the cellular constituents of the pulmonary arteries. Investigators have reported evidence of proliferative, apoptosis-resistant, cancer-like behavior in endothelial cells, SMCs, and fibroblasts from subjects with PAH [89–91]. Specific observations leading to this concept include monoclonal expansion of endothelial cells from patients with iPAH when compared to patients with PAH associated with congenital heart disease, instability of short DNA microsatellite sequences within plexiform lesions, somatic chromosome abnormalities in the lungs of patients with PAH, persistent hyperproliferative and apoptosis-resistant state when endothelial cells are removed from their in vivo environment, and altered energy metabolism [92]. Enhanced proliferation of pulmonary vascular cells may be a consequence of excessive growth factor release from the ECM, alterations in growth factor production or receptor expression, and/or alterations in intracellular mitogenic signals [93–95]. Abnormal increases in key apoptotic factors including Bcl-xL, Bcl-2, and survivin have been reported in pulmonary vascular cells from PAH patients [58, 96, 97]. Although there is evidence of enhanced cell proliferation and resistance to apoptosis, vascular remodeling in PAH is distinguished from cancer in that there is no evidence that pulmonary vascular cells have the ability to reproduce in a clonal fashion without control.

RISK FACTORS

Older age of onset
Longstanding duration of disease > 5 years
Anti-centromere antibody
Anti-nuclear antibody nucleolar pattern
Anti-U1 RNP antibody
Absence of anti-Scl 70 antibody
DLCO < 60% predicted
FVC %predicted/DLCO %predicted > 1.6
Elevated N-terminal pro BNP

PAH GENETIC MUTATIONS

BMPR2 - bone morphogenetic protein receptor 2
ALK1 - activin receptor like kinase type 1
CAV1 - caveolin 1
ENG - endoglin
KKCNK3 - potassium channel super family K member 3
SMAD4 - acronym from fusion of *Caenorhabditis elegans*
SMAD9 *Sma* genes and the *Drosophila Mad*

SSC-PAH GENETIC MUTATIONS

TNFAIP3 - tumor necrosis factor alpha induced protein 3
TLR2 - Toll like receptor 2
uPAR - urokinase type plasminogen activator receptor
CAV1 - caveolin 1

ENDOTHELIAL DYSFUNCTION

Excessive endothelin-1 production
Deficiency of nitric oxide production
Deficiency of prostacyclin production
Excessive thromboxane production

SMOOTH MUSCLE CELL DYSFUNCTION

Impaired potassium channel ($K_{V1.5}$) function

OTHER PATHOGENETIC MECHANISMS

Inflammation, Cytokines and Growth Factors
- Inflammatory cell infiltrates in vascular lesions
- Elevated Interleukins 1 beta, 2, 4, 6, 8 10 and 12p70
- Elevated TNF- alpha, CXC3L1, CCL2, CCL 5
- PDGF

Epigenetic mechanisms
- DNA methylation
- Histone modification
- Micro RNAs

Autoantibodies
- Anti-endothelial cell antibodies
- Anti-fibroblast antibodies

Cancer-like cell characteristics
- Monoclonal expansion of endothelial cells in iPAH
- Unstable short DNA microsatellite sequences
- Somatic chromosome abnormalities
- Hyperproliferation/apoptosis resistance ex vivo
- Metabolic shift from glucose oxidation to glycolysis

Serotonin
- SMC and fibroblast proliferation

Table 2.
Summary of factors involved in pathogenesis of pulmonary arterial hypertension.

Endothelial cells, SMCs, and adventitial fibroblasts from patients with PAH are not only more proliferative and apoptosis-resistant but rely more on glycolysis for energy production [89, 98–100]. Mitochondria demonstrate a metabolic shift from glucose oxidation to uncoupled aerobic glycolysis similar to that described in cancer cells [101]. The glycolytic pathway increases NADPH production which in turn enhances antioxidant defenses while producing ribonucleotides for DNA synthesis. This shift in metabolism serves as a mechanism to support rapid cell proliferation.

3.3.7 Ion channels

Increased cytosolic calcium levels in SMCs of patients with PAH promote not only contraction but also hyperproliferation and apoptosis resistance [41]. Elevated cytosolic Ca^{+2} levels in PAH have been linked to downregulation of voltage-gated potassium channels, such as Kv1.5 [102]. Downregulation or dysfunction of voltage-gated potassium channels allows membrane depolarization and influx of calcium. Cytosolic calcium levels are further enhanced by impaired mitochondrial Ca^{+2} uptake. The resulting increases in intracellular calcium drive cells into the cell cycle, thus enhancing proliferation [103].

Research has certainly revealed that the pathogenesis of PAH is a very complex process, and our understanding of the mechanisms involved is far from complete. Knowledge of imbalances in endogenously produced vasomotor regulators has allowed the development of therapies that have improved quality of life and survival. However, it is apparent that PAH is not merely a disease of vasomotor dysfunction, but one that involves complex genetic mechanisms, cytokines, inflammation, and metabolic derangements (**Table 2**). While the progressive arteriopathy of iPAH and SSc-PAH shares many features, research has disclosed distinct differences in the pathogenesis of the two entities that may lead to more effective treatments for each in the future.

4. Screening and diagnosis

The majority of patients with SSc-PAH are diagnosed with PAH when the pulmonary arteriopathy is well established, while a small percentage is diagnosed at an early, asymptomatic stage [2]. Even when symptoms are present, the symptoms of PAH are nonspecific and may be attributed to other causes. Mortality is higher in patients with SSc-PAH than iPAH or PAH associated with other disease processes, such as congenital heart disease [104, 105]. An estimated 1-year survival of 84% for patients with iPAH contrasts with a 55% rate of survival at 1 year in SSc-PAH [106]. Patients with SSc-PAH have a higher mortality rate than those with non-scleroderma connective tissue disease-associated PAH [107]. Further, mortality is higher in patients with SSc- PAH than in systemic sclerosis patients without lung involvement or with lung involvement other than PAH [108]. In recent years, PAH and lung fibrosis have replaced scleroderma renal crisis as major causes of death in systemic sclerosis [109]. Pulmonary arterial hypertension accounts for about 30% of deaths in systemic sclerosis [109, 110]. Three-year survival rates of 70, 50, and 20% have been reported in treated SSc-PAH patients with WHO FC 1, FC 2, and FC 3 symptoms, respectively [107]. Earlier discovery of PAH in the systemic sclerosis patient may have an impact on these discouraging survival statistics. In a study by Humbert et al., the 1-, 3-, 5-, and 8-year survival rates in a cohort of SSc-PAH patients managed according to routine practice were 75%, 31%, 25%, and 17%, respectively, compared to survival rates of 100%, 81%, 73%, and 64%, respectively, in a group managed in a proactive detection program [111]. These data underscore the importance of consistently screening patients with systemic sclerosis for PAH.

Although experts agree on the importance of screening for SSc-PAH in order to detect vascular involvement at an earlier stage, there is less consensus on the most effective algorithm to confirm the presence of PAH. Several risk factors have been identified that signal the potential for the development of SSc-PAH (**Table 2**). Patients who are older and have long-standing SSc are at greater risk of developing PAH [1, 112]. The limited cutaneous form of SSc has historically been considered a risk for PAH; however the presence of diffuse cutaneous SSc has also been reported with similar prevalence [13, 113]. Anticentromere antibodies (ACA), anti-U1-ribonucleoprotein antibodies (RNP), and a nucleolar pattern of antinuclear antibody (nucleolar-ANA) are associated with an increased risk of SSc-PAH [114–117]. The absence of anti-Scl 70 has been associated with the development of PAH, while the presence of these autoantibodies is associated with the development of interstitial lung disease [14]. Symptoms that relate to PAH are nonspecific and typically relate to progressive right ventricular (RV) dysfunction. Common symptoms include shortness of breath, fatigue, weakness, chest pain, and syncope [118]. Physical findings suggesting PAH include an accentuated pulmonary component of the second heart sound, an RV third heart sound, a pansystolic murmur of tricuspid regurgitation, and a diastolic murmur of pulmonary regurgitation [16]. Jugular venous distension, hepatomegaly, ascites, edema, and cyanosis are findings in advanced disease. Certain findings on electrocardiogram, such as right axis deviation, RV hypertrophy, RV strain, and right bundle branch block, may point to a diagnosis of PAH. Electrocardiogram abnormalities are more likely to be found in severe PAH. A normal electrocardiogram does not exclude PAH. Plain chest radiography can also be helpful in diagnosing PAH if the X-ray demonstrates central pulmonary artery enlargement, pruning of the peripheral vessels, or enlargement of right heart chambers. A chest radiograph may be helpful in distinguishing other causes of PH if interstitial lung disease or pulmonary venous congestion is present. Similarly, pulmonary function tests can be very helpful in detecting airway disease or restrictive lung disease that could lead to WHO Group 3 PH. Pulmonary function testing in patients with SSc-PAH may reveal severe gas diffusion impairment. Mukerjee et al. noted that a DLCO <50% was 90% specific but only 39% sensitive in excluding a diagnosis of SSc-PAH [6]. A DLCO/VA <70% or FVC percent/DLCO percent >1.6 has been considered predictors for the development of SSc-PAH [119]. Pulmonary function testing and CXR or high-resolution CT scanning are helpful in distinguishing PAH from WHO Group 3 PH associated with ILD. Echocardiography has been considered a noninvasive alternative to RHC in determining the presence of SSc-PAH, although certain limitations are recognized. Factors affecting image quality have been noted to limit the ability to estimate pulmonary artery systolic pressure accurately in patients who were later confirmed to have PAH by RHC [120, 121]. Right heart catheterization is the gold standard for diagnosis of PAH and is required to confirm PAH. Right heart catheterization with saline volume challenge can be helpful in distinguishing WHO Group 2 PH due to abnormal left ventricular function in systemic sclerosis. Several algorithms have been proposed that rely on various combinations of symptoms, physical exam findings, biomarkers, PFTs, and findings on echocardiography to determine which patients warrant definitive study with right heart catheterization [10, 16, 120, 122, 123].

A screening algorithm including assessment of symptoms, Doppler echocardiography, and right heart catheterization was studied in a French prospective multicenter study by the Itinerair-Scleroderma Investigators Group that enrolled 599 patients with scleroderma [120]. The study was limited to patients without significant pulmonary function abnormalities. Patients with a velocity of tricuspid regurgitation (VTR) > 3 m/s regardless of symptoms and patients with a VTR 2.5–3 m/s with dyspnea were considered at risk for PAH and underwent right heart catheterization (RHC). Right heart catheterization confirmed mild PAH in 18 of 33 patients suspected of having PAH based on symptoms and/or Doppler echocardiography. Twelve of the 33 patients did not have PAH, and 3 patients were confirmed to have left heart dysfunction. This algorithm allowed early detection of SSc-PAH; however a substantial number of patients undergoing RHC did not have PAH.

An alternative screening algorithm was suggested by the Australian Scleroderma Interest Group (ASIG) that employs N-terminal pro-brain natriuretic peptide (NT-proBNP) levels and PFT data to predict the presence of PAH [122]. Data to develop this algorithm were collected from the Australian Scleroderma Cohort Study, a multicenter study of risk and prognostic factors for cardiopulmonary outcomes in systemic sclerosis. NT-proBNP levels from SSc patients with confirmed PAH were compared with a group at risk for PAH (systolic $PAP_{TTE} > 36$ mmHg, hemoglobin corrected DLCO <50% predicted, and/or FVC/DLCO percent predicted ≥1.6), a group with ILD, and a group of controls with no evidence of cardiopulmonary complications. NT-proBNP levels were positively correlated with systolic PAP by transthoracic echocardiogram, mean PAP by RHC, pulmonary vascular resistance, and mean right atrial pressure. The authors proposed a model in which patients screened positive when NT-proBNP was ≥209.8 pg./ml and/or DLCO was <70.3% with FVC/DLCO ≥1.82. They noted a sensitivity of 100% with specificity 77.8% for SSc-PAH but acknowledged a need for prospective validation of the model.

A third screening algorithm was employed in the DETECT study, a multinational, cross-sectional investigation of factors in SSc patients that could serve to detect PAH at an earlier stage [10]. A broad range of variables (112 in total) pertaining to standard demographic and clinical characteristics, serum tests, electrocardiography, and echocardiography were examined in patients with a diagnosis of systemic sclerosis for more than 3 years, a predicted DLCO <60%, and a predicted FVC ≥ 40%. About 466 patients underwent RHC and 87 (19%) were confirmed to have WHO Group 1 PAH. Univariate and multivariate analyses were used to select the variables with best discriminatory power for predicting PAH. These variables

Resting echocardiography is recommended as a screening test in asymptomatic patients with systemic sclerosis.
A combined approach (including biomarkers, PFTs and echocardiography) should be considered to predict PH in systemic sclerosis.
Initial screening using the stepwise DETECT algorithm may be considered in adult systemic sclerosis patients with > 3 years disease duration and a DLCO < 60% predicted.
Annual screening with echocardiography, PFTs and biomarkers may be considered in patients with systemic sclerosis.
Systemic sclerosis patients with a mean PAP ranging from 21 to 24 mmHg should be closely monitored, because of a higher risk of PAH.
Exercise echocardiography is not recommended to predict PH in high risk populations.

Adapted from: Galie N, Humbert M, Vachiery J-L et al. 2015 ESC/ERS Guidelines for the diagnosis and treatment of pulmonary hypertension. Eur Heart J 2016; 37(1): 67-119

Table 3.
2015 ESC/ERS recommendations for pulmonary arterial hypertension screening in systemic sclerosis.

were incorporated in a two-step algorithm. Six non-echocardiographic variables were used in Step 1 to recommend echocardiography (FVC % predicted/DLCO % predicted, current/past telangiectasias, serum anti-centromere antibody, NT-pro BNP, serum urate, ECG with right axis deviation), and a decision to recommend RHC in Step 2 was based on right atrial area and velocity of tricuspid regurgitation (VTR). Complete Step 1 data were available for 356 patients. About 52 patients did not meet Step 1 criteria for referral to echocardiography. Of these, two patients (4%) were determined to be false PAH negative. Complete Step 2 data were available for 267 patients. About 69 patients did not meet Step 2 criteria for referral to RHC. Of these, one patient was determined to be false PAH negative. Of the 198 patients referable for RHC, 69 were true PAH positive. The overall sensitivity of this algorithm was 96% with a specificity of 48%, a 62% rate of referral for RHC, and a 4% false PAH negative rate.

Summary recommendations for PAH screening in systemic sclerosis from the 2015 European Society of Cardiology/European Respiratory Society (ESC/ERS) Guidelines for the Diagnosis and Treatment of Pulmonary Hypertension are summarized in **Table 3**. The guidelines support a combined approach incorporating biomarkers, PFTs, and echocardiography for baseline screening in patients with systemic sclerosis. Annual screening with these indicators should be considered for all patients with systemic sclerosis. Systemic sclerosis patients with a mean PAP from 21 to 24 mmHg should continue to be monitored closely for progression. Exercise echocardiography has been used for early detection of PAH in systemic sclerosis [124, 125]; however the ESC/ERS do not recommend this approach. A summary diagnostic algorithm is provided in **Figure 3**.

5. Treatment

As understanding of the pathogenesis of PAH has evolved over the past two decades, a number of medical therapies have been developed that improve exercise capacity, hemodynamics, quality of life, and survival. Treating PAH has become a complex exercise now that there are multiple agents that can be employed alone or in various combinations. It is important to remember that PAH is a progressive disease process, and any treatment plan requires ongoing monitoring and adjustment if treatment goals are not being met. Although far fewer patients with PAH require lung transplantation in the era of targeted medical therapy, there are those who progress even on maximal medical therapy leaving transplantation as their last viable option.

The treatment of pulmonary arterial hypertension involves not only selection of appropriate agents for inclusion in a treatment plan but an ongoing process of assessment of patient characteristics that should determine the selection of medications. The concept of using a risk assessment tool to aid selection of appropriate agents for treatment was introduced in 2006 based on studies showing correlation between clinical characteristics of disease and survival [104]. For instance, 6 MW, FC, and certain hemodynamic measures were shown to directly correlate with prognosis. These findings were used to develop a tool to evaluate a patient's risk of early death. Patients could be categorized as low or high risk of rapid progression to death, and treatment agents could be selected based on the level of risk in order to modify the course of disease and extend survival. This concept further evolved with the development of a risk calculator using data from the American REVEAL Registry [126, 127]. The REVEAL Registry was a 3-year longitudinal registry of 2967 WHO Group 1 PAH patients with data collected pertaining to the clinical characteristics, evaluation, treatment, and outcomes. Data from this registry was used to develop a user-friendly algorithm to determine a patient's risk of demise in the short term. Most recently, the ESC/ERS further refined the characteristics used to assess risk of progression in PAH and presented criteria that classified patients as low, moderate, or high risk of progression to near-term death (**Figure 2**). Using the ESC/ERS risk assessment algorithm, patients categorized as low risk have an estimated 1-year mortality <5%. Those within the intermediate-risk group have an estimated 1-year mortality of 5–10%, and those in the high-risk group have an estimated 1-year mortality >10%.

5.1 Risk assessment

Following the accurate diagnosis of PAH (**Figure 3**), a careful assessment of severity of disease should be completed before deciding on specific treatment options. This assessment is critical at the outset of treatment, but it remains an important part of ongoing patient management. Given that PAH can progress rapidly, even on therapy, it is necessary to complete a reevaluation of severity of illness and risk stratification periodically several times a year. If patients show signs of deterioration in their clinical parameters, treatment plan adjustments are in order.

5.1.1 Functional capacity

Assessment of the severity of illness begins with an understanding of symptoms and functional capacity. Patients who present symptoms, such as shortness of breath, fatigue, or edema, that have developed and worsened over a short period of time are at higher risk of early death. Further, those with overt signs of right heart failure, such as edema, ascites, cyanosis, or syncope, are in a high-risk group requiring urgent attention. The World Health Organization functional class (FC) is a valuable indicator of severity of illness and has been shown to correlate with survival [128, 129]. Patients are classified in four groups (FC 1–4) based on degree

Determinant of prognosis	Low Risk <5%	Intermediate Risk 5-10%	High Risk >10%
Clinical signs of right heart failure	Absent	Absent	Present
Progression of symptoms	No	Slow	Rapid
Syncope	No	Occasional [a]	Repeated [b]
WHO functional class	I, II	III	IV
6 MW distance	> 440 m	165-440 m	< 165 m
Cardiopulmonary exercise testing	Peak VO_2 > 15 ml/min/kg (> 65% predicted) VE/VCO_2 slope <36	Peak VO_2 11-15 ml/min/kg (35-65% pred) VE/VCO_2 slope 36-44.9	Peak VO_2 <11 ml/min/kg (< 35 % predicted) VE/VCO_2 slope ≥45
NT-proBNP level	BNP < 50 ng/l NT-proBNP <300 ng/l	BNP 50-300 ng/l NT-proBNP 300-1400 ng/l	BNP > 300 ng/l NT-proBNP >1400 ng/l
Imaging by echocardiogram or cardiac MRI	RA area <18 cm^2 No pericardial effusion	RA area 18-26 cm^2 No or minimal pericardial effusion	RA area >26 cm^2 Pericardial effusion
Hemodynamics	RAP <8 mmHg CI > 2.5 l/min/m^2 SvO_2 >65%	RAP 8-14 mmHg CI 2.0-2.4 l/min/m^2 SvO_2 60-65%	RAP >14 mmHg CI < 2.0 l/min/m^2 SvO2 < 60%

ESC/ERS= European Society of Cardiology/European Respiratory Society; WHO= World Health Organization; 6 MW= 6 minute walk; VO_2= oxygen consumption; VE/VCO_2 = ventilatory equivalents for carbon dioxide; NT-proBNP= N-terminal pro brain natriuretic peptide; BNP= brain natriuretic peptide; MRI= magnetic resonance imaging; RA= right atrium; RAP= right atrial pressure; CI= cardiac index; SvO_2= mixed venous oxygen saturation
[a] occasional syncope with brisk or heavy exercise or occasionally orthostatic syncope
[b] repeated episodes of syncope regardless of activity level

Adapted from Galie N, Humbert M, Vachiery J-L et al. 2015 ESC/ERS Guidelines for the diagnosis and treatment of pulmonary hypertension. Eur Heart J 2016; 37(1): 67-119.

Figure 2.
ESC/ERS risk assessment in pulmonary arterial hypertension (estimated risk for 1-year mortality).

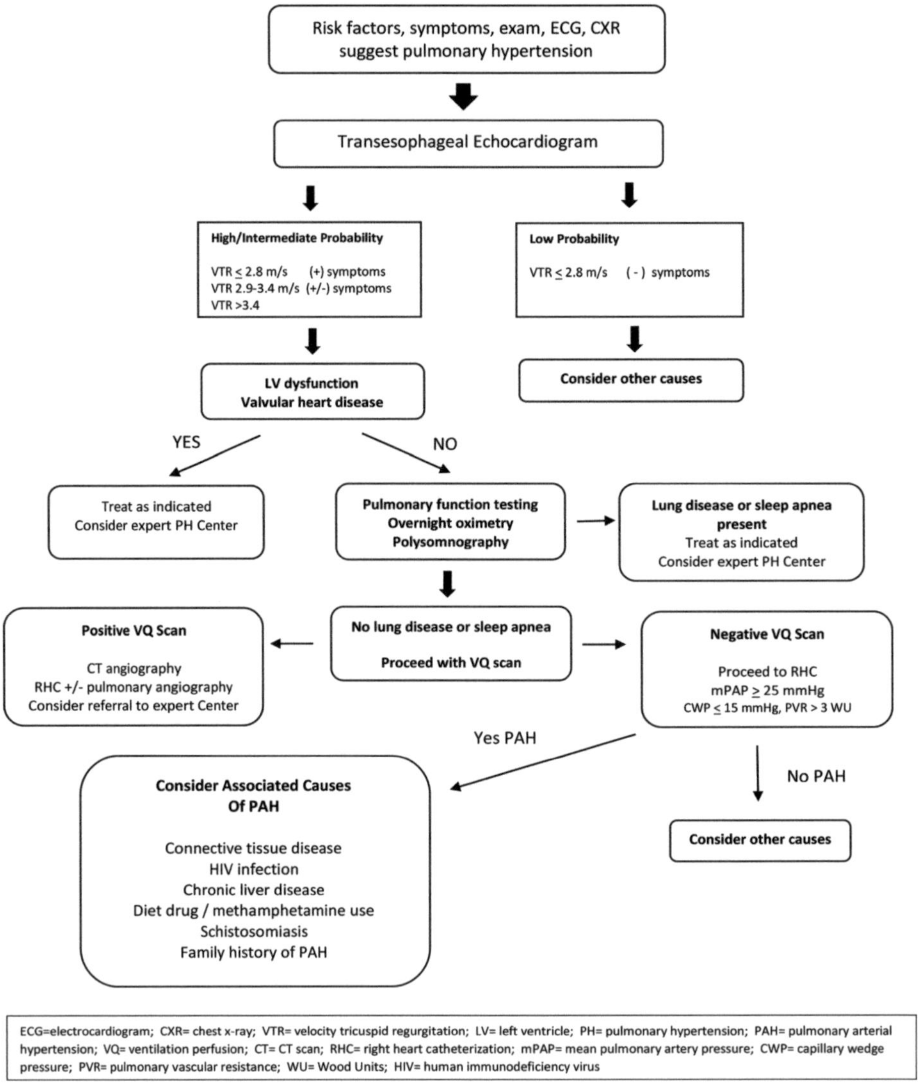

Figure 3.
Algorithm for the diagnosis of pulmonary arterial hypertension.

of functional impairment (**Table 4**). Patients who have FC 3 or 4 functional impairment are considered high risk; a goal of any treatment plan is to achieve FC 1 or 2 functional capacity [16]. Although functional class has been shown to correlate well with survival prognosis, it is a subjective measure of symptoms which is subject to interpretation by the healthcare provider [130]. Another important indicator of illness severity is the 6 min walk (6 MW) test [131]. The 6 MW test is a submaximal exercise test that is easy to perform in the outpatient or inpatient setting. The 6 MW test has been shown to correlate with survival and has served as a primary endpoint in the majority of clinical investigations leading to today's therapeutic options [132, 133]. Six-min walk distance has been shown to correlate with pulmonary pressures and represent a direct predictor of mortality in SSc-PAH [131]. The ESC/ERS Guidelines suggest that patients who can ambulate >440 m have better survival prognosis and are an appropriate goal to target when making treatment decisions [16]. The 6 MW test does have limitations with its reliability being challenged by factors such as age, gender, weight, comorbid conditions, and the individual's

Class	Funtional capacity
I	Patient with pulmonary hypertension but without resulting limitations of physical activity. Ordinary physical activity does not cause undue fatigue or dyspnea, chest pain, or syncope.
II	Patient with pulmonary hypertension resulting in slight limitation of physical activity. Patient is comfortable at rest. Ordinary physical activity results in fatigue or dyspnea, chest pain or syncope.
III	Patient with pulmonary hypertension resulting in marked limitation of physical activity. Patient is comfortable at rest. Less than ordinary physical activity causes undue fatigue or dyspnea, chest pain or syncope.
IV	Patient with pulmonary hypertension resulting in inability to carry on any physical activity without symptoms. Patient with signs of right heart failure. Dyspnea and/or fatigue may occur even at rest.

Table 4.
The World Health Organization (WHO) functional class.

motivation. Cardiopulmonary exercise testing (CPET) is often employed to evaluate exercise capacity in this population. CPET can provide important information about general exercise capacity, as well as more detailed information about gas exchange, ventilation, and cardiac function during exercise. Patients with PAH will demonstrate exercise limitation characterized by low end-tidal partial pressure of carbon dioxide (pCO_2), high ventilation equivalents for carbon dioxide (VE/VCO_2), low oxygen pulse (VO_2/HR), and low peak oxygen uptake (peak VO_2) [134, 135]. These parameters have been included in the ESC/ERS risk assessment algorithm. Peak VO_2 > 15 ml/min/kg or greater than 65% predicted and a VE/VCO_2 slope < 36 portend a more favorable prognosis and represent goals of targeted therapy [136].

5.1.2 Echocardiography and hemodynamics

Echocardiography is not only a valuable screening tool for detecting the presence of pulmonary hypertension, but it plays a role in assessing severity of illness and response to treatment. The measurement of pulmonary artery pressure (PAP) by echocardiography is not a reliable prognostic indicator, nor does it accurately reflect progression or improvement in pulmonary vascular resistance [121, 128]. The absence of tricuspid regurgitation and/or poor image quality limits the ability to determine systolic PAP by echocardiography in 20–39% of patients [121]. The value of echocardiography in assessing severity of illness lies in measurement of chamber sizes, assessment of right ventricular (RV) function, and the presence or absence of pericardial effusion which is considered a reflection of RV failure. A complete echocardiographic assessment in the PAH patient would include description of right atrial (RA) and RV dimensions, measurement of tricuspid regurgitant velocity, left ventricular (LV) eccentricity index, and RV contractility [137, 138]. RV contractility can be determined from RV longitudinal systolic strain/strain rate, RV fractional area change, Tei index, or tricuspid annular plane systolic excursion (TAPSE) [137, 139]. Echocardiography with exercise may provide useful information about RV function. An increase in estimated PAP by >30 mmHg during exercise indicates better RV reserve associated with better long-term outcome and is considered an independent marker of prognosis in PAH [140]. A right atrial area < 18 cm^3 with no evident pericardial effusion are indicators for favorable prognosis or treatment outcome [16]. Additional information about prognosis or treatment effect can be gained from right heart catheterization and hemodynamic measurements. As in the case of echocardiography, PA pressure is of little value. Cardiac index, RA pressure, and mixed venous oxygen saturation have been shown to have the greatest prognostic significance [128, 129]. Goals of therapy that are associated with favorable prognosis include CI ≥ 2.5 L/min/m^2, RA pressure < 8 mmHg, and SvO2 > 65% [16].

5.1.3 Biomarkers

There are a number of biomarkers of vascular dysfunction, inflammation, cardiac function, and tissue hypoxia that have been investigated as a specific marker for pulmonary vascular remodeling [141–144]. Of these, brain natriuretic peptide (BNP) and NT-proBNP are used in clinical practice and research [145–147]. These biomarkers reflect ventricular wall stress, as seen in volume overload and ventricular contractile dysfunction, and serve as surrogate indicators of myocardial dysfunction [122, 148]. Either marker is considered an acceptable choice for assessing severity of illness. BNP has slightly better correlation with pulmonary vascular hemodynamics and is less likely to be affected by renal function, while NT-proBNP appears to be a stronger predictor of prognosis [149]. Compared to BNP, NT-proBNP is more sensitive to early increases in systolic PAP as measured by echocardiography [150]. BNP levels below 50 ng/L or NT-proBNP levels below 300 ng/L are associated with a more favorable prognosis [16].

5.1.4 Monitoring

Implementation of the prognostic indicators outlined in **Figure 2** is variable among centers providing expert care for patients with PAH. After a treatment plan is established, patients will typically be reevaluated every 3–4 months depending on stability of their disease. During early phases of treatment or times when therapy targets indicate a need to alter the treatment plan, patients are often seen more frequently. It is not practical to perform all of the measures listed in **Figure 3** at every visit. In the outpatient setting, clinicians tend to rely on assessment of symptoms, physical exam findings, FC, 6 MW distance, and BNP or NT-proBNP levels to determine severity of disease at any given point in time. This information may be supplemented periodically with echocardiography or cardiopulmonary exercise testing. Right heart catheterization is performed initially at diagnosis and in some centers yearly thereafter or in the event condition deteriorates in those patients with high-risk features. In other centers repeat hemodynamic measurements are obtained less frequently and typically if there is an indication the patient's condition is progressing.

Once the diagnosis is established and severity of illness is defined, decisions about disease-targeted therapy can be made. Available targeted therapies exert clinical benefit via the nitric oxide, endothelin, or prostacyclin pathways which were discussed earlier in this chapter. There are several options that affect each of these pathways. The choice of therapy for any given patient will depend on severity of illness and may be further influenced by side effects, safety issues, and in some cases economic and social support factors.

5.2 Phosphodiesterase 5 inhibitors

The phosphodiesterase 5 (PDE-5) inhibitors effect smooth muscle relaxation and inhibit proliferation and inflammatory mechanisms by augmenting cyclic guanosine monophosphate (cGMP) activity in pulmonary vascular smooth muscle. As noted earlier in this chapter, patients with PAH have been shown to have deficient nitric oxide synthase activity in the pulmonary vasculature leading to a deficiency of nitric oxide production [54]. Nitric oxide is produced by the pulmonary endothelium and catalyzes the production of cGMP in nearby smooth muscle cells. PDE-5 degrades cGMP, thus limiting its effect on smooth muscle cells. The phosphodiesterase 5 inhibitors sildenafil and tadalafil block the degradation of cGMP, thus permitting beneficial cGMP effects to continue.

5.2.1 Sildenafil

Sildenafil has been shown to improve symptoms, exercise capacity, and hemodynamics in patients with PAH including those with connective tissue disease (CTD) [151, 152]. It is available as an oral agent prescribed at 20 mg tid. This drug is generally well tolerated with most common side effects including headache, flushing, nausea, and nasal congestion, all resulting from vasodilation. The use of nitroglycerin is contraindicated in patients taking sildenafil due to a risk of severe hypotension when these drugs are used in combination. Safety during human pregnancy has not been studied; however no fetal harm has been noted in animal studies.

5.2.2 Tadalafil

Tadalafil has also proven to have beneficial effects on symptoms, exercise capacity, hemodynamics, and time to clinical worsening in a large randomized clinical trial involving 405 PAH patients including 95 with connective tissue disease [153]. Tadalafil's greatest benefit was realized at a dose of 40 mg daily. The drug is well tolerated with side effects and precautions similar to sildenafil.

5.2.3 Vardenafil

Vardenafil is a third agent within the PDE-5 inhibitor class that demonstrated significant advantage when comparing 6 MW distance, cardiac index, mean PA pressure, and pulmonary vascular resistance in patients treated with vardenafil 5 mg twice daily or placebo [154]. The long-term effects of vardenafil in PAH have not been evaluated, and the drug has not been approved for the treatment of PAH in the United States.

5.3 Soluble guanylate cyclase stimulators

While the phosphodiesterase 5 inhibitors promote vasodilation and limit proliferation by preventing the degradation of cGMP, the soluble guanylate cyclase (sGC) stimulator riociguat interacts directly with guanylate cyclase to stimulate production of cGMP [54].

5.3.1 Riociguat

Riociguat is the only member of this family in use to date. Riociguat was studied in two randomized clinical trials, one focused on patients with PAH (PATENT 1) and included those with CTD [155] and the other patients with chronic thromboembolic pulmonary hypertension (CTEPH) [156]. Significant improvements were observed in exercise capacity, FC, time to clinical worsening, and hemodynamics. Subgroup analysis of the PATENT 1 trial specifically evaluating benefit in CTD-PAH revealed improvements in 6 MW, FC, pulmonary vascular resistance, and cardiac index [157]. Riociguat is an oral therapy with maximum daily use of 2.5 mg tid. Side effects are similar to those seen with the PDE-5 inhibitors. In addition, riociguat can induce systemic hypotension and has been linked to an increased risk of bleeding. It is teratogenic and contraindicated in pregnancy. Females of childbearing age are required to participate in a Risk Evaluation and Mitigation Strategy (REMS) program and undergo monthly pregnancy testing in addition to practicing careful contraceptive measures. This drug should not be used with nitroglycerin or PDE-5 inhibitors due to the risk of severe hypotension.

5.4 Endothelin receptor antagonists

Excessive levels of endothelin 1 produced by pulmonary vascular endothelial cells have been implicated in the vasoconstriction and cell proliferation seen in PAH [57, 158, 159]. Endothelin binds with two G protein-coupled receptors, type A and B, located on the smooth muscle cell surface and thereby promotes its physiologic effects. Type A receptors mediate vasoconstriction, cell growth, and inflammation, while type B receptors mediate opposing effects including vasodilation and natriuresis while inhibiting proliferation and inflammation.

5.4.1 Bosentan

Bosentan was the first targeted oral therapy developed to treat PAH and is prescribed with a bid dosing schedule. Bosentan has been investigated in patients with iPAH, PAH associated with CTD, and Eisenmenger syndrome [160–162]. The drug interacts with both type A and B receptors to effect improvements in exercise capacity, FC, time to clinical worsening, hemodynamics, and echocardiographic variables [163]. About 10% of patients treated with bosentan in clinical trials developed reversible elevations in liver transaminases. Monthly monitoring of liver function tests is required for patients using bosentan. Other side effects that can be seen are fluid retention and anemia. Further, this drug is teratogenic and contraindicated during pregnancy. Females of childbearing age who use bosentan must enroll in a Risk Evaluation and Mitigation Strategy (REMS) program and are required to undergo monthly pregnancy testing. They should be counseled to avoid pregnancy with careful contraceptive practices if sexually active. It is important to note that hormonal contraceptive effectiveness is reduced by bosentan. It is also important to note that cyclosporine and glyburide may increase bosentan levels and increase the risk of liver toxicity.

5.4.2 Ambrisentan

Ambrisentan is a selective endothelin type A receptor blocker which is available as an oral therapy prescribed for once daily use. This drug has been studied in one pilot and two randomized clinical trials demonstrating improvements in symptoms, exercise capacity, time to clinical worsening, and hemodynamics in patients with iPAH, CTD-PAH, and HIV-associated PAH [164, 165]. The risk of liver function abnormalities is minimal, and monthly liver function testing is not required for patients using ambrisentan; however its use is not recommended in patients with moderate to severe liver dysfunction. Ambrisentan use can be complicated by the development of edema and anemia. Like bosentan, ambrisentan is teratogenic and contraindicated during pregnancy. All of the precautions relating to use in females of childbearing age noted for bosentan are also true for ambrisentan.

5.4.3 Macitentan

Macitentan is the most recent endothelin 1 antagonist available to PAH patients as a once daily oral therapy. Like bosentan, macitentan is a dual endothelin receptor blocker. In contrast to bosentan and ambrisentan, the benefits of macitentan were realized in a large event-driven investigation involving 742 patients treated for an average of 100 weeks [166]. Macitentan significantly reduced time from initiation to a composite endpoint of worsening PAH, initiation of intravenous or subcutaneous prostanoid therapy, atrial septostomy, lung transplantation, or death. The study population included a significant proportion of patients on background therapy who also experienced significant benefit. Macitentan is well tolerated and, as with other endothelin antagonists, may be associated with fluid retention or anemia. Again, this drug is teratogenic and contraindicated during pregnancy. Patients using this drug should follow the same risk reduction recommendations as noted with bosentan and ambrisentan.

5.5 Prostacyclin analogues

A deficiency of prostacyclin activity characterizes the dysfunction of the third major pathway involved in the development of PAH. Prostacyclin is produced by the pulmonary endothelium, and its bioactive effects include vasodilation of the pulmonary vascular bed, inhibition of platelet aggregation, and cell proliferation [167]. A reduction of prostacyclin synthase expression has been recognized in pulmonary arteries from patients with PAH and is thought to be the central focus of dysfunction in this pathway [55]. The prostacyclin analogues are available as oral, inhaled, or systemically administered disease-targeted therapies.

5.5.1 Epoprostenol

Epoprostenol is available for use as a continuous intravenous (IV) infusion. Epoprostenol has a short half-life of 3–5 min. The original formulation was unstable at room temperature after about 8 h and required considerable effort to maintain at cooler temperatures. A newer formulation of the drug is now available that has extended room temperature stability. Treatment is initiated at a dose of 2–4 ng/kg/min and titrated upward to reach clinical therapy targets. Patients experience tachyphylaxis with the continuous infusion, therefore requiring intermittent dose escalation over time. The maximum beneficial dose of epoprostenol is typically 40 ng/kg/min, although titration may go beyond this point. Epoprostenol has been shown to improve symptoms, exercise capacity, and hemodynamics in FC 3 and 4 patients with iPAH and SSc-PAH [168–170]. Side effects with epoprostenol can be pronounced and may include jaw pain, nausea, diarrhea, flushing, and headache. There is a risk of catheter-related complications including infection and thrombosis. Epoprostenol can cause hypotension when used with other antihypertensives and may increase risk of bleeding when used in patients taking anticoagulants or antiplatelet agents. Epoprostenol has been used during pregnancy without evidence of fetal harm to date. Given the short half-life of epoprostenol, an infusion of this drug should not be discontinued abruptly due to the risk of rebound pulmonary vasoconstriction and death.

5.5.2 Treprostinil

Treprostinil is an analogue of epoprostenol available in systemic, inhaled, and oral formulations. The systemically infused form of treprostinil is stable at room temperature, has a half-life of 3–4 h, and can be administered by continuous subcutaneous (SC) or IV infusions. Dosing typically begins with 1–2 ng/kg/min with gradual dose escalation to achieve clinical target goals. Side effects are similar to epoprostenol. Additionally those patients using the subcutaneous formulation may experience significant infusion site pain. Several topical analgesic preparations are available that can successfully control local infusion site pain. As is the case with epoprostenol, patients develop tachyphylaxis requiring dose escalation to maintain clinical benefit. The usual effective dose is 20–80 ng/kg/min, although dosing can extend well beyond this range. Treprostinil was first studied in its continuous SC formulation. A randomized clinical trial of 470 patients treated with SC treprostinil, including 17% CTD patients, revealed improvements in exercise tolerance and hemodynamics [171, 172]. Dose titration was limited by side effects, including infusion site pain, and as such benefits were noted in those patients achieving higher doses >13.8 ng/kg/min. Later treprostinil was approved for use as a continuous IV infusion. Treprostinil can be administered in an inhaled formulation with a specialized nebulizer four times daily. This formulation is very well tolerated with most commonly reported effects including mouth soreness, cough, and headache. Tachyphylaxis does not develop due to intermittent dosing. Some patients may notice recurrence of PAH symptoms as effect wanes between treatments. In a randomized clinical trial of inhaled treprostinil added to background therapy with bosentan or sildenafil, there were improvements in 6 MW, NT-proBNP levels, and quality of life measures [173]. More recently, treprostinil has been offered in an oral formulation that is taken by either bid or tid scheduled dosing. Although intermittent dosing is employed in the treatment of patients with oral treprostinil, dose escalation over time helps achieve and maintain clinical target goals. The use of oral treprostinil can be complicated by significant gastrointestinal side effects, such as nausea, anorexia, and diarrhea. In a randomized clinical trial of treatment-naïve PAH patients, oral treprostinil use was associated with improvement in 6 MW distance [174]. Treprostinil can cause hypotension when used with other antihypertensives and may increase risk of bleeding when used in patients taking anticoagulants or antiplatelet agents. Parenteral and inhaled treprostinil safety during pregnancy has not been studied in humans but did not lead to fetal harm in animals, and as such they have Category B designations. Oral treprostinil has been associated with adverse fetal effects in animal studies and is designated Category C. Continuous IV therapy carries a risk of catheter-related complications including infection and thrombosis. Oral treprostinil use is contraindicated in patients with Child-Pugh Class 3 hepatic impairment. Treprostinil should not be discontinued abruptly due to the risk of rebound pulmonary vasoconstriction and death.

5.5.3 Iloprost

Iloprost is a stable analogue of prostacyclin that is also available in IV, inhaled, or oral formulations. Oral iloprost has not been evaluated for use; however, both the IV and inhaled forms have been used in Europe, and the inhaled form has been approved for use in the United States. The inhaled formulation is administered with a specifically designed handheld and portable nebulizer device. This form of iloprost is used by nebulization 6–9 times a day at a dose of 2.5–5 ug/inhalation. The effect lasts from 30 to 90 min. The intermittent dosing eliminates the development of tachyphylaxis. Improvements in symptoms, exercise capacity, and pulmonary vascular resistance were observed in a clinical trial in which iloprost was compared with placebo in patients with PAH and CTEPH [175]. The effect of IV iloprost was noted to be similar to epoprostenol in a small group of patients with PAH and CTEPH [176]. The inhaled drug is well tolerated with most frequent side effects being cough, flushing, and jaw pain. Inhaled iloprost can cause hypotension and should be avoided or used cautiously in patients with relative hypotension.

5.6 Prostacyclin receptor agonist

The development of the prostacyclin receptor agonist class of disease-targeted therapies represents a new approach to treating PAH. Although the prostacyclin receptor agonism of this new class is similar to that of prostacyclins, the receptor interaction is selective for the IP receptor. The established prostanoid receptors in the human pulmonary artery are the IP, EP_3, and TP receptors. The IP receptor mediates vasodilation and inhibits proliferation, while the EP_3 and TP receptors may promote vasoconstriction and cell proliferation [177–179].

5.6.1 Selexipag

Selexipag is a selective IP receptor agonist that is structurally distinct from prostacyclin with an active metabolite that is 37-fold more potent. Selexipag is prescribed for oral BID dosing beginning with 200 mcg bid and titrating to a maximal dose of up to 1600 mcg bid. The target treatment dose for individual patients is determined by the development of side effects limiting further dose escalation. Selexipag reduced the risk of reaching a composite morbidity and mortality (worsening PAH resulting in need for atrial septostomy or lung transplantation, initiation of parenteral prostanoid therapy or chronic oxygen therapy, hospitalization for PAH, other indication of disease progression, or death) by 40% in a large placebo-controlled, event-driven trial including 1156 patients [180, 181]. At baseline, 80% of patients were being treated with stable doses of an endothelin blocker, a PDE-5 inhibitor, or both. A subgroup analysis of 334 patients with connective tissue disease-associated PAH (170 SSc, 82 systemic lupus, 82 mixed or other) revealed a similar 41% reduction in risk of the composite morbidity and mortality events [182]. Further the treatment effect was consistent regardless of background PAH treatment or connective tissue disease subtype. Commonly reported side effects include headache, nausea, diarrhea, flushing, myalgia, and arthralgia.

5.7 Combination therapy

Despite observations from clinical trials that individual therapeutic agents can improve exercise capacity, time to clinical worsening, and hemodynamics, pulmonary arterial hypertension remains a progressive disease that is difficult to control. The progressive nature of this disease process in patients treated with monotherapy has fostered the practice of combining agents to limit progression. One approach has been the sequential addition of agents affecting the three known pathophysiologic pathways. In this approach an agent affecting one of the pathways is chosen to begin monotherapy and if clinical response is inadequate, one or more agents affecting the other pathways are added until desired clinical benefit is achieved. Upfront combination therapy has become a more contemporary approach to managing pulmonary arterial hypertension. This approach to treating PAH was conceived from experience with the treatment of other disease states, such as cancer or congestive heart failure, with agents affecting multiple mechanisms of disease upfront. The upfront combination approach gained momentum with the AMBITION trial which demonstrated a 50% reduction in composite morbidity/mortality events in patients treated with an upfront combination of tadalafil and ambrisentan compared to either agent as monotherapy [183]. This benefit was also recognized in a subgroup analysis of patients with CTD-PAH and SSc-PAH [184].

Hemodynamics, RV structure and function, and overall functional status were significantly improved in SSc-PAH patient treated with the upfront combination [185]. Investigations of several newer treatments for PAH, such as riociguat, macitentan, and selexipag, have included significant proportions of patients on background therapies and have demonstrated added improvements in exercise capacity, functional class, and time to clinical worsening [155, 166, 181]. These studies have fueled the impetus to include recommendations for combination therapy in contemporary treatment guidelines [16, 186].

5.8 Nonmedical treatment options

Medical therapy can improve activity tolerance, hemodynamics, and quality of life and can even improve survival prognosis; however, in some cases PAH will progress even with aggressive medical therapy. Nonmedical options may include balloon atrial septostomy and/or lung transplantation. Atrial septostomy may be beneficial in FC 4 patients with right heart failure or severe syncopal symptoms who are progressing on maximal medical therapy [187]. Atrial septostomy is also a consideration as a bridge to lung transplantation when medical therapy fails. An interatrial right-to-left shunt may decompress the right heart chambers and ultimately improve oxygen transport despite an observed oxyhemoglobin desaturation [188]. Atrial septostomy is not recommended in end-stage patients with mean RAP >20 mmHg and a resting room air saturation below 85% [187, 188]. Lung transplantation is also an option for patients with end-stage SSc-PAH failing medical therapy. In some centers, patients with SSc-PAH may not be offered lung transplantation due to the risk of aspiration pneumonia related to esophageal disease. However, studies have shown that survival after lung transplantation is similar in patients with SSc-PAH and other transplant indications [189]. There has been increasing interest in stem cell therapy as a treatment option for PAH. Although animal models have shown some promise, stem cell therapy is not currently a viable option for treatment of human PAH [190].

5.9 Treatment algorithm

The poor survival prognosis associated with SSc-PAH and the availability of multiple disease-targeted treatment options have fostered the development of algorithms to guide the treatment decision process. Both the American College of Chest Physicians [186] and the Joint Task Force for the Diagnosis and Treatment of Pulmonary Hypertension of the ESC/ERS [16] have published guidelines to aid clinicians in the treatment of patients with PAH.

5.10 Supportive measures

In addition to a careful risk assessment, choice of appropriate disease-targeted agent, and close monitoring of treatment effect, there are severe supportive measures that apply in the management of the patient with SSc-PAH. Patients are not restricted from physical activity. Physical activity and supervised rehabilitation have been shown to improve exercise tolerance, reduce fatigue, and improve quality of life [191, 192]. The ESC/ERS Guidelines suggest that patients who are stable clinically should consider participation in a rehabilitation program at a center experienced with the management of PAH if possible [16]. Patients with SSc-PAH should be vaccinated against influenza and pneumococcal pneumonia. Pregnancy in patients with PAH is associated with a high mortality risk and should be avoided. If patients with PAH become pregnant, the high risk of complications and pregnancy termination should be discussed. Some PAH treatments cause fetal harm, and patients are required to undergo monthly pregnancy monitoring when using such therapies. Riociguat and the endothelin antagonists are teratogenic. Patients using these targeted therapies should be carefully counseled about the risk of fetal harm and instructed to use at least two barrier methods of contraception while using these agents. In the event patients do become pregnant, they may continue PAH therapies that are not considered fetal toxic, such as the prostanoids, plan an elective delivery, and work closely with a high-risk obstetrical team and experienced pulmonary hypertension specialist throughout the pregnancy [193]. Patients with PAH are often overwhelmed by the physical limitations, financial burden, and social impact associated with PAH [194]. Screening for depression is helpful in identifying patients who could benefit from referral to appropriate services in the community where help is available to ease the psychosocial burden of this disease. Genetic counseling may be appropriate for select patients [195]. It is often helpful for the affected patient and at-risk family members to understand their mutation status in order to plan for the future. Genetic testing and counseling should involve a multidisciplinary team including pulmonary hypertension specialists, genetic counselors, geneticists, psychologists, and nurses. Elective surgery is not contraindicated but does carry an increased risk to the PAH patient. Patients with significantly impaired RV function are at highest risk and should undergo careful preoperative assessment [196–198]. Epidural anesthesia may be better tolerated [199]. Patients using oral therapies may require transition to an intravenous or inhaled form of therapy until able to take oral medications postoperatively.

6. Conclusions

Pulmonary arterial hypertension is a leading cause of death in patients with systemic sclerosis. While the pathogenesis of PAH in the patient with systemic sclerosis bears resemblance to that of idiopathic PAH, there are distinct differences in genetic predisposition, role of inflammation and autoantibodies, and pathologic manifestations of disease. Early detection is essential in preventing early demise from SSc-PAH. Several algorithms have been suggested for screening SSc patients for PAH. In general, it is recommended that annual screening with biomarkers, PFTs, and echocardiography be considered in any patient with systemic sclerosis, even if they are asymptomatic. There are a number of medical therapies available which have demonstrated benefit in SSc-PAH, as well as iPAH. The importance of regular monitoring and repeat risk assessment cannot be underemphasized. Lung transplantation may be an option for those patients who progress on maximal medical therapy. While the prognosis for SSc-PAH has certainly improved over the past two decades, continued research into the mechanisms of disease and development of new treatments will ensure further improvements in quality of life and survival in the future.

Author details

John W. Swisher[1]* and Shashank Kailash[2]

1 East Tennessee Pulmonary Hypertension Center, Fort Sanders Regional Medical Center, Knoxville, TN, USA

2 Department of Medicine, Brandon Regional Hospital, Brandon, FL, USA

*Address all correspondence to: jswisher@statcaremed.net

References

[1] Avouac J, Airo P, Meune C, et al. Prevalence of pulmonary hypertension in systemic sclerosis in European Caucasians and meta-analysis of 5 studies. The Journal of Rheumatology. 2010;**37**(11):2290-2298

[2] Varga J, Steen V. Pulmonary arterial hypertension in systemic sclerosis (scleroderma): Definition, classification, risk factors, screening, and prognosis. UpToDate. 2018

[3] Hao Y, Thakkar V, Stevens W, et al. A comparison of the predictive accuracy of three screening models for pulmonary arterial hypertension in systemic sclerosis. Arthritis Research and Therapy. 2015;**17**:7-18

[4] Iudici M, Codullo V, Giuggioli D, et al. Pulmonary hypertension in systemic sclerosis: prevalence, incidence and predictive factors in a large multicentric Italian cohort. Clinical and Experimental Rheumatology. 2013;**31**(Suppl 76):31-36

[5] Murata I, Kihara H, Shinohara S, et al. Echocardiographic evaluation of pulmonary arterial hypertension in patients with systemic and related syndromes. Japanese Circulation Journal. 1992;**56**:983-991

[6] Mukerjee D, St George D, Coleiro B, et al. Prevalence and outcome in systemic sclerosis associated pulmonary arterial hypertension: application of a registry approach. Annals of the Rheumatic Diseases. 2003;**62**:1088-1093

[7] Yang X, Mardekian J, Sanders KN, et al. Prevalence of pulmonary arterial hypertension in patient with connective tissue diseases: A systematic review of the literature. Clinical Rheumatology. 2013;**32**:1519-1531

[8] Niklas K, Niklas A, Mularek-Kubzdela T, et al. Prevalence of pulmonary hypertension in patients with systemic sclerosis and mixed connective tissue disease. Medicine. 2018;**97**(28):e11437

[9] Morrisroe K, Stevens W, Sahhar J, et al. Epidemiology and disease characteristics of systemic sclerosis-related pulmonary arterial hypertension: Results from a real-life screening programme. Arthritis Research and Therapy. 2017;**19**:42

[10] Coghlan JG, Denton CP, Grunig V, et al. Evidence-based detection of pulmonary arterial hypertension in systemic sclerosis: The DETECT study. Annals of the Rheumatic Diseases. 2014;**73**:1340-1349

[11] Hinchcliff M, Fischer A, Schiopu E, et al. Pulmonary hypertension assessment and recognition of outcomes in scleroderma (PHAROS): Baseline characteristics and description of study population. The Journal of Rheumatology. 2011;**38**(10):2172-2179

[12] Chang B, Schachna L, White B, et al. Natural history of mild-moderate pulmonary hypertension and the risk factors for severe pulmonary hypertension in scleroderma. The Journal of Rheumatology. 2006;**33**(2):269-274

[13] Cox SR, Walker JG, Coleman M, et al. Isolated pulmonary hypertension in scleroderma. Internal Medicine Journal. 2005;**35**(1):28-33

[14] Steen V, Medsger TA Jr. Predictors of isolated pulmonary hypertension in patients with systemic sclerosis and limited cutaneous involvement. Arthritis and Rheumatism. 2003;**48**(2):516-522

[15] Simmoneau G, Gatzoulis M, Adatia I, et al. Updated clinical classification of pulmonary hypertension. Journal of

the American College of Cardiology. 2013;**62**:D34-D41

[16] Galie N, Humbert M, Vachiery J-L, et al. 2015 ESC/ERS Guidelines for the diagnosis and treatment of pulmonary hypertension. European Heart Journal. 2016;**37**(1):67-119

[17] Tuder RM, Marcki JC, Richter A, et al. Pathology of pulmonary hypertension. Clinics in Chest Medicine. 2007;**28**(1):23-42

[18] Gaine S. Pulmonary hypertension. Journal of the American Medical Association. 2000;**284**:3160-3168

[19] Tuder RM, Ponticos M, Holmes A. Pathogenesis of pulmonary arterial hypertension. In: Varga J et al., editors. Scleroderma. New York, NY: Springer Science; 2017. pp. 385-401

[20] Chazova I, Loyd JE, Newman JH, et al. Pulmonary artery adventitial changes and venous Involvement in primary pulmonary hypertension. The American Journal of Pathology. 1999;**146**:389-397

[21] Ishibashi-Ueda H, Ohta-Ogo K. Human pathology. In: Fukumoto Y, editor. Diagnosis and Treatment of Pulmonary Hypertension. Singapore: Springer; 2017

[22] Cool CD, Kennedy D, Voelkel NF, et al. Pathogenesis and evolution of plexiform lesions in pulmonary hypertension associated with scleroderma and human immunodeficiency virus infection. Human Pathology. 1997;**28**(4):434-442

[23] Foshat M, Boroumand N. The evolving classification of pulmonary hypertension. Archives of Pathology and Laboratory Medicine. 2017;**141**:696-703

[24] Atkinson C, Stewart S, Upton PD, et al. Primary pulmonary hypertension is associated with reduced pulmonary vascular expression of type II bone morphogenetic protein receptor. Circulation. 2002;**105**(4):1672-1678

[25] Tuder RM, Zaiman AL. Pathology of pulmonary vascular disease. In: Peacock A, Rubin LJ, editors. Pulmonary Circulation. London: Hodder Arnold, Health Sciences; 2003

[26] Sakao S, Taraseviciene-Stewart L, Lee JD, et al. Initial apoptosis is followed by increased proliferation of apoptosis-resistant endothelial cells. The FASEB Journal. 2005;**19**(9):1178-1180

[27] Palevsky HI, Schloo BL, Peitra GG, et al. Primary pulmonary hypertension, vascular structure, morphometry, and responsiveness to vasodilator agents. Circulation. 1989;**80**:1207-1221

[28] Balk AG, Dingemans KP, Wagenvoort CA. The ultrastructure of the various forms of pulmonary arterial intimal fibrosis. Virchows Archiv. A, Pathological Anatomy and Histology. 1979;**382**:139-150

[29] Stenmark KR, Davie N, Frid M, et al. Role of the adventitia in pulmonary vascular remodeling. Physiology. 2006;**21**:134-145

[30] Bou-Gharios G, Ponticos M, Rajkumar V, et al. Extra-cellular matrix in vascular networks. Cell Proliferation. 2004;**37**:207-220

[31] Nagase H, Visse R, Murphy G. Structure and function of matrix metalloproteinases and TIMPS. Cardiovascular Research. 2006;**69**:562-573

[32] Safdar Z, Tamez E, Chan W, et al. Circulating collagen biomarkers as indicators of disease severity in pulmonary arterial hypertension. JACC: Heart Failure. 2014;**2**:412-421

[33] Wang Z, Lakes RS, Golob M, et al. Changes in large pulmonary arterial viscoelasticity in chronic pulmonary hypertension. PLoS One. 2013;**8**:e78569

[34] Golledge J, Clancy P, Maguire J, et al. The role of tenascin C in cardiovascular disease. Cardiovascular Research. 2011;**92**:19-28

[35] Wei L, Warburton RR, Preston IR, et al. Serotonylated fibronectin is elevated in pulmonary hypertension. American Journal of Physiology. Lung Cellular and Molecular Physiology. 2012;**302**:L1273-L1279

[36] Stacher E, Graham BB, Hunt JM, et al. Modern age pathology of pulmonary arterial hypertension. American Journal of Respiratory and Critical Care Medicine. 2012;**186**:261-272

[37] Argula RG, Harley RA, Silver RM, et al. The differences between systemic sclerosis associated pulmonary arterial hypertension (ssc-Pah) and idiopathic pulmonary arterial hypertension (ipah): A quantitative lung morphometric analysis. American Journal of Respiratory and Critical Care Medicine. 2017;**195**:A7404

[38] Overbeek MJ, Vonk MC, Boonstra A, et al. Pulmonary arterial hypertension in limited cutaneous systemic sclerosis: A distinctive vasculopathy. The European Respiratory Journal. 2009;**34**:371-379

[39] Deng Z, Morse JH, Slager SL, et al. Familial primary pulmonary hypertension (gene PPH1) is caused by mutations in the bone morphogenetic protein receptor II gene. American Journal of Human Genetics. 2000;**67**:737-744

[40] Lane KB, Machado RD, Pauciulo MW, et al. Heterozygous germline mutations in BMPR2, encoding a TGF-beta receptor, cause familial primary pulmonary hypertension. Nature Genetics. 2000;**26**:81-84

[41] Thenappan T, Ormiston ML, Ryan JJ, et al. Pulmonary arterial hypertension: Pathogenesis and clinical management. British Medical Journal. 2018;**360**:j5492

[42] Broen JC, Bossini-Castillo L, van Bon L, et al. A rare polymorphism in the gene for toll-like receptor 2 is associated with systemic sclerosis phenotype and increases the production of inflammatory mediators. Arthritis and Rheumatism. 2012;**64**:264-271

[43] Dieude P, Guedj M, Wipff J, et al. Association of TNFAIP3 rs 5029939 variant with systemic sclerosis in the European Caucasian population. Annals of the Rheumatic Diseases. 2010;**69**:1958-1964

[44] Manetti M, Allanore Y, Revillod L, et al. A genetic variation located in the promoter region of the UPAR (CD87) gene is associated with the vascular complications of systemic sclerosis. Arthritis and Rheumatism. 2011;**63**:247-256

[45] Austin ED, Loyd JE. The genetics of pulmonary arterial hypertension. Circulation Research. 2014;**115**:189-202

[46] Morrell NW, Yang X, Upton PD, et al. Altered growth responses of pulmonary artery smooth muscle cells from patients with primary pulmonary hypertension to transforming growth factor-beta(1) and bone morphogenetic proteins. Circulation. 2001;**104**:790-795

[47] Good RB, Gilbane AJ, Trinder SL, et al. Endothelial to mesenchymal transition contributes to endothelial dysfunction in pulmonary artery hypertension. The American Journal of Pathology. 2015;**185**:1850-1858

[48] Varga J, Whitfield ML. Transforming growth factor-beta

in systemic sclerosis (scleroderma). Frontiers in Bioscience (Scholar Edition). 2009;**1**:226-235

[49] Upton PD, Davies RJ, Tajsic T, et al. Transforming growth factor-beta(1) represses bone morphogenetic protein-mediated Smad signaling in pulmonary artery smooth muscle cells via Smad 3. American Journal of Respiratory Cell and Molecular Biology. 2013;**49**:1135-1145

[50] Davies RJ, Holmes AM, Deighton J, et al. BMP type II receptor deficiency confers resistance to growth inhibition by TGF-beta in pulmonary artery smooth muscle cells; role of proinflammatory cytokines. American Journal of Physiology. Lung Cellular and Molecular Physiology. 2012;**302**:L604-L615

[51] Burton VJ, Ciuclan LI, Holmes AM, et al. Bone morphogenetic protein receptor II regulates pulmonary artery endothelial cell barrier function. Blood. 2011;**117**:333-341

[52] Derrett-Smith EC, Dooley A, Gilbane AJ, et al. Endothelial injury in a transforming growth factor beta-dependent mouse model of scleroderma induces pulmonary arterial hypertension. Arthritis and Rheumatism. 2013;**65**:2928-2939

[53] Gilbane AJ, Derrett-Smith E, Trinder SL, et al. Impaired bone morphogenetic protein receptor II signaling in a transforming growth factor-beta-dependent mouse model of pulmonary hypertension in systemic sclerosis. American Journal of Respiratory and Critical Care Medicine. 2015;**191**:665-677

[54] Giaid A, Saleh D. Reduced expression of endothelial nitric oxide synthase in the lungs of patients with pulmonary hypertension. The New England Journal of Medicine. 1995;**333**:214-221

[55] Tuder RM, Cool CD, Geraci MW, et al. Prostacyclin synthase expression is decreased in lungs from patients with severe pulmonary hypertension. American Journal of Respiratory and Critical Care Medicine. 1999;**159**:1925-1932

[56] Christman B, McPherson C, Newman J, et al. An imbalance between the excretion of thromboxane and prostacyclin metabolites in pulmonary hypertension. The New England Journal of Medicine. 1992;**327**:70-75

[57] Giaid A, Yanagisawa M, Langleban D, et al. Expression of endothelin-1 in the lungs of patients with pulmonary hypertension. The New England Journal of Medicine. 1993;**328**:1732-1739

[58] McMurtry MS, Archer SL, Altieri DC, et al. Gene therapy targeting surviving selectively induces pulmonary vascular apoptosis and reverses pulmonary arterial hypertension. The Journal of Clinical Investigation. 2005;**115**:1479-1491

[59] Tuder RM, Chacon M, Alger LA, et al. Expression of angiogenesis-related molecules in plexiform lesions in severe pulmonary hypertension: Evidence for a process of disordered angiogenesis. The Journal of Pathology. 2001;**195**:367-374

[60] Achar RO, Demura Y, Rai PR, et al. Loss of caveolin and heme oxygenase expression in severe pulmonary hypertension. Chest. 2006;**129**:696-705

[61] MacLean MR, Herve P, Eddahibi S, et al. 5-hydroxytryptamine and the pulmonary circulation: Receptors, transporters and relevance to pulmonary arterial hypertension. British Journal of Pharmacology. 2000;**131**:161-168

[62] Welsh DJ, Harnett M, MacLean M, et al. Proliferation and signaling in fibroblasts: Role of 5-hydroxytryptamine2A receptor

and transporter. American Journal of Respiratory and Critical Care Medicine. 2004;**170**:252-259

[63] Lee SL, Wang WW, Lanzillo JJ, et al. Serotonin produces both hyperplasia and hypertrophy of bovine pulmonary artery smooth muscle cells in culture. The American Journal of Physiology. 1994;**266**:L46-L52

[64] Ren W, Watts SW, Fanburg BL. Serotonin transporter interacts with the PDGFbeta receptor in PDGF-BB-induced signaling and mitogenesis in pulmonary artery smooth muscle cells. American Journal of Physiology. Lung Cellular and Molecular Physiology. 2011;**300**:L486-L497

[65] Dees C, Akhmetshina A, Zerr P, et al. Platelet-derived serotonin links vascular disease and tissue fibrosis. The Journal of Experimental Medicine. 2011;**208**:961-972

[66] Seibold JR, Molony RR, Turkevich D, et al. Acute hemodynamic effects of ketanserin in pulmonary hypertension secondary to systemic sclerosis. The Journal of Rheumatology. 1987;**14**:519-524

[67] Kim GH, Ryan JJ, Marsboom G, et al. Epigenetic mechanisms of pulmonary hypertension. Pulmonary Circulation. 2011;**1**:347-356

[68] Wang Y, Kahaleh B. Epigenetic repression of bone morphogenetic protein receptor II expression in scleroderma. Journal of Cellular and Molecular Medicine. 2013;**17**:1291-1299

[69] Zhao L, Chen CN, Hajji N, et al. Histone deacetylation inhibition in pulmonary hypertension: Therapeutic potential of valproic acid and suberoylanilide hydroxamic acid. Circulation. 2012;**126**:455-467

[70] Kim J, Kang Y, Kojima Y, et al. An endothelial apelin-FGF link mediated by miR-424 and miR-503 is disrupted in pulmonary arterial hypertension. Nature Medicine. 2013;**19**:74-82

[71] Heath D, Yacoub M. Lung mast cells in plexogenic pulmonary arteriopathy. Journal of Clinical Pathology. 1991;**44**:1003-1006

[72] Perros F, Dorfmuller P, Souza R, et al. Dendritic cell recruitment in lesions of human and experimental pulmonary hypertension. The European Respiratory Journal. 2007;**29**:462-468

[73] Humbert M, Monti G, Brenot F, et al. Increased interleukin-1 and interleukin-6 serum concentrations in severe primary pulmonary hypertension. American Journal of Respiratory and Critical Care Medicine. 1995;**151**:1628-1631

[74] Soon E, Holmes AM, Treacy CM, et al. Elevated levels of inflammatory cytokines predict survival in idiopathic and familial pulmonary arterial hypertension. Circulation. 2010;**122**:920-927

[75] Perros F, Dorfmuller P, Souza R, et al. Fractalkine-induced smooth muscle cell proliferation in pulmonary hypertension. The European Respiratory Journal. 2007;**29**:937-943

[76] Sanchez O, Marcos E, Perros F, et al. Role of endothelium-derived CC chemokine ligand 2 in idiopathic pulmonary arterial hypertension. American Journal of Respiratory and Critical Care Medicine. 2007;**176**:1041-1047

[77] Dorfmuller P, Zarka V, Durand-Gasselin I, et al. Chemokine RANTES in severe pulmonary arterial hypertension. American Journal of Respiratory and Critical Care Medicine. 2002;**165**:534-539

[78] Tuder RM, Groves BM, Badesch DB, et al. Exuberant endothelial cell

growth and elements of inflammation are present in plexiform lesions of pulmonary hypertension. American Journal of Respiratory and Critical Care Medicine. 1994;**144**:275-285

[79] El Kasmi KC, Pugliese SC, Riddle SR, et al. Adventitial fibroblasts induce a distinct proinflammatory/profibrotic macrophage phenotype in pulmonary hypertension. Journal of Immunology. 2014;**193**:597-609

[80] Savai R, Pullamsetti SS, Kolbe J, et al. Immune and inflammatory cell involvement in the pathology of idiopathic pulmonary arterial hypertension. American Journal of Respiratory and Critical Care Medicine. 2012;**186**:897-908

[81] Perros F, Dorfmuller P, Montani D, et al. Pulmonary lymphoid neogenesis in idiopathic pulmonary arterial hypertension. American Journal of Respiratory and Critical Care Medicine. 2012;**185**:311-321

[82] Antoniu SA. Targeting PDGF pathway in pulmonary arterial hypertension. Expert Opinion on Therapeutic Targets. 2012;**16**:1055-1063

[83] Overbeek MJ, Boonstra A, Voskuyl AE, et al. Platelet-derived growth factor receptor-beta and epidermal growth factor receptor in pulmonary vasculature of systemic sclerosis-associated pulmonary arterial hypertension versus idiopathic pulmonary arterial hypertension and pulmonary veno-occlusive disease: A case control study. Arthritis Research and Therapy. 2011;**13**:R61

[84] Frost AE, Barst RJ, Hoeper MM, et al. Long-term safety and efficacy of imatinib in pulmonary arterial hypertension. The Journal of Heart and Lung Transplantation. 2015;**34**:1366-1375

[85] Tamby MC, Chanseaud Y, Humbert M, et al. Anti-endothelial cell antibodies in idiopathic and systemic sclerosis associated pulmonary arterial hypertension. Thorax. 2005;**60**:765-772

[86] Dib H, Tamby MC, Bussone G, et al. Targets of anti-endothelial cell antibodies in pulmonary hypertension and scleroderma. The European Respiratory Journal. 2012;**39**:1405-1414

[87] Li M, Ai J, Tian Z, et al. Prevalence of anti-endothelial cell antibodies in patients with pulmonary arterial hypertension associated with connective tissue diseases. Chinese Medical Sciences Journal. 2010;**25**:27-31

[88] Tamby MC, Humbert M, Guilpain P, et al. Antibodies to fibroblasts in idiopathic and scleroderma-associated pulmonary hypertension. The European Respiratory Journal. 2006;**28**:799-807

[89] Archer SL, Gomberg-Maitland M, Maitland ML, et al. Mitochondrial metabolism, redox signaling, and fusion: A mitochondria-ROS-HIF-1alpha-Kv1.5 O_2-sensing pathway at the intersection of pulmonary hypertension and cancer. American Journal of Physiology. Heart and Circulatory Physiology. 2008;**294**:H570-H578

[90] Caruso P, Dunmore BJ, Schlosser K, et al. Identification of miR-124 as a major regulator of enhanced endothelial cell glycolysis in pulmonary arterial hypertension via PTBP1 and PKM2. Circulation. 2017;**136**(25):2451-2467

[91] Zhang H, Wang D, Li M, et al. The metabolic and proliferative state of vascular adventitial fibroblasts in pulmonary hypertension is regulated through a miR-124/PTBP1/PKM axis. Circulation. 2017;**136**(25):2468-2485

[92] Guignabert C, Tu L, LeHiress M, et al. Pathogenesis of pulmonary arterial hypertension: lessons. from cancer. European Respiratory Review. 2013;**22**:543-551

[93] Izikki M, Guignabert C, Fadel E, et al. Endothelial-derived FGF2 contributes to the progression of pulmonary hypertension in humans and rodents. The Journal of Clinical Investigation. 2009;**119**:512-523

[94] Merklinger SL, Jones PL, Martinez EC, et al. Epidermal growth factor receptor blockade mediates smooth muscle cell apoptosis and improves survival in rats with pulmonary hypertension. Circulation. 2005;**112**:423-431

[95] Schermuly RT, Dony E, Ghofrani HA, et al. Reversal of experimental pulmonary hypertension by PDGF inhibition. Journal of Clinical Investigation. 2005;**115**:2811-2821

[96] Tu L, De Man FS, Girerd B, et al. A critical role for p130Cas in the progression of pulmonary hypertension in humans and rodents. American Journal of Respiratory and Critical Care Medicine. 2012;**186**:666-676

[97] Tu L, Dewachter L, Gore B, et al. Autocrine fibroblast factor-2 signaling contributes to altered endothelial phenotype in pulmonary hypertension. American Journal of Respiratory Cell and Molecular Biology. 2011;**45**:311-322

[98] Xu W, Koeck T, Lara AR, et al. Alterations of cellular bioenergetics in pulmonary artery endothelial cells. Proceedings of the National Academy of Sciences of the United States of America. 2007;**104**:1342-1347

[99] Tuder RM, Davis LA, Graham BB. Targeting energetic metabolism: A new frontier in the pathogenesis and treatment of pulmonary hypertension. American Journal of Respiratory and Critical Care Medicine. 2012;**185**:260-266

[100] Sutendra G, Michelakis ED. The metabolic basis of pulmonary arterial hypertension. Cell Metabolism. 2014;**19**:558-573

[101] Ryan JJ, Archer SL. Emerging concepts in the molecular basis of pulmonary arterial hypertension: Part 1: Metabolic plasticity and mitochondrial dynamics in the pulmonary circulation and right ventricle in pulmonary arterial hypertension. Circulation. 2015;**131**:1691-1702

[102] Yuan X-J, Wang J, Juhaszova M, et al. Attenuated K channel gene transcription in primary pulmonary hypertension. Lancet. 1998;**351**:726-727

[103] Yuan JX, Aldinger AM, Juhaszova M, et al. Dysfunctional voltage-gated K^+ channels in pulmonary artery smooth muscle cells of patients with primary pulmonary hypertension. Circulation. 1998;**98**:1400-1406

[104] McLaughlin VV, McGoon MD. Pulmonary arterial hypertension. Circulation. 2006;**114**:1417-1431

[105] Simeon-Aznar CP, Fonollasa-Pla V, Tolosa-Vilella C, et al. Registry of the Spanish network for systemic sclerosis: Survival, prognostic factors, and causes of death. Medicine (Baltimore). 2015;**94**:e1728

[106] Kawut SM, Taichman DB, Archer Chicko CL, et al. Hemodynamics and survival in patients with pulmonary arterial hypertension related to systemic sclerosis. Chest. 2003;**123**:344-350

[107] Condliffe R, Kiely DG, Peacock AJ, et al. Connective tissue disease-associated pulmonary arterial hypertension in the modern treatment era. American Journal of Respiratory and Critical Care Medicine. 2009;**179**:151-157

[108] Koh ET, Lee P, Gladman DD, et al. Pulmonary hypertension in systemic sclerosis: An analysis of 17 patients. British Journal of Rheumatology. 1996;**35**:989-993

[109] Steen VD, Medsger TA. Changes in causes of death in systemic sclerosis,

1972-2002. Annals of the Rheumatic Diseases. 2007;**66**:940-944

[110] Tyndall AJ, Bannert B, Bonk M, et al. Causes and risk factors for death in systemic sclerosis: A study from the EULAR Scleroderma Trials and Research (EUSTAR) database. Annals of the Rheumatic Diseases. 2010;**69**:1809-1815

[111] Humbert M, Azzedine Y, De Groote P, et al. Screening for pulmonary arterial hypertension in patients with systemic sclerosis. Arthritis and Rheumatism. 2011;**63**:3522-3530

[112] Schchna L, Wigley FM, Chang B, et al. Age and risk of pulmonary arterial hypertension in scleroderma. Chest. 2003;**124**:2098

[113] Hunzelmann N, Genth E, Krieg T, et al. The registry of the German Network for Systemic Scleroderma: Frequency of disease subsets and patterns of organ involvement. Rheumatology. 2008;**47**:1185-1192

[114] Steen VD. Autoantibodies in systemic sclerosis. Seminars in Arthritis and Rheumatism. 2005;**35**:35-42

[115] Kampolis C, Plastiras S, Vlachoyiannopoulos P, et al. The presence of anti-centromere antibodies may predict progression of estimated pulmonary arterial systolic pressure in systemic sclerosis. Scandinavian Journal of Rheumatology. 2008;**37**:278-283

[116] Aggarwal R, Lucas M, Fertig N, et al. Anti-U3 RNP autoantibodies in systemic sclerosis. Arthritis and Rheumatology. 2009;**60**:1112-1118

[117] Assous N, Allanore Y, Batteux F, et al. Prevalence of antiphospholipid antibodies in systemic sclerosis and association with primitive pulmonary arterial hypertension and endothelial injury. Clinical and Experimental Rheumatology. 2005;**23**:199-204

[118] McLaughlin VV, Archer SL, Badesch DB, et al. ACCF/AHA expert consensus document on pulmonary hypertension. Journal of the American College of Cardiology. 2009;**53**:1573-1619

[119] Allanore Y, Borderie D, Avouac J, et al. High N-terminal pro-brain natriuretic peptide levels and low diffusing capacity for carbon monoxide as independent predictors of the occurrence of precapillary pulmonary arterial hypertension in patients with systemic sclerosis. Arthritis and Rheumatism. 2008;**58**:284-291

[120] Hachulla E, Gressin V, Guillevin L, et al. Early detection of pulmonary arterial hypertension in systemic sclerosis: A French nationwide prospective multicenter study. Arthritis and Rheumatism. 2005;**52**:3792-3800

[121] Denton CP, Cailes JB, Phillips GD, et al. Comparison of doppler echocardiography and right heart catheterization to assess pulmonary hypertension in systemic sclerosis. British Journal of Rheumatology. 1997;**36**:239-243

[122] Thakkar V, Stevens WM, Prior D, et al. N-terminal pro-brain natriuretic peptide in a novel screening algorithm for pulmonary arterial hypertension in systemic sclerosis: A case control study. Arthritis Research and Therapy. 2012;**14**:R143

[123] Khanna D, Gladue H, Channick R, et al. Recommendations for screening and diagnosis of connective-tissue disease associated pulmonary arterial hypertension. Arthritis and Rheumatism. 2013;**65**. DOI: 10.1002/art.38172

[124] Nagel C, Henn P, Ehlken N, et al. Stress doppler echocardiography for early detection of systemic sclerosis-associated pulmonary arterial

hypertension. Arthritis Research and Therapy. 2015;**17**:165

[125] Baptista R, Serra S, Martins R, et al. Exercise echocardiography for the assessment of pulmonary hypertension in systemic sclerosis: A systematic review. Arthritis Research and Therapy. 2016;**18**:153

[126] Benza RL, Gomberg-Maitland M, Miller DP, et al. The REVEAL registry risk score calculator in patients newly diagnosed with pulmonary arterial hypertension. Chest. 2012;**141**:354-362

[127] McGoon MD, Miller DP. REVEAL: A contemporary US pulmonary arterial hypertension registry. European Respiratory Review. 2012;**21**:8-18

[128] Nickel N, Golpon H, Greer M, et al. The prognostic impact of follow-up assessments in patients with idiopathic pulmonary arterial hypertension. The European Respiratory Journal. 2012;**39**:589-596

[129] Benza RL, Miller DP, Gomberg-Maitland M, et al. Predicting survival in pulmonary arterial hypertension: Insights from the Registry to Evaluate Early and Long-Term Pulmonary Arterial Hypertension disease management (REVEAL). Circulation. 2010;**122**:164-172

[130] Taichman DB, McGoon MD, Harhay MO, et al. Wide variation in clinicians' assessment of New York Heart Association/World Health Organization functional class in patient with pulmonary arterial hypertension. Mayo Clinic Proceedings. 2009;**84**:586-592

[131] Gadre A, Ghattas C, Han X, et al. Six-minute walk test as a predictor of diagnosis, disease severity, and clinical outcomes in scleroderma-associated pulmonary hypertension: The DIBOSA study. Lung. 2017;**195**:529-536

[132] Savarese G, Paolillo S, Costanzo P, et al. Do changes in 6-minute walk distance predict clinical events in patients with pulmonary arterial hypertension?: A meta-analysis of 22 randomized trials. Journal of the American College of Cardiology. 2012;**60**:1192-1201

[133] Gabler NB, French B, Strom BL, et al. Validation of 6-minute walk distance as a surrogate end point in pulmonary arterial hypertension trials. Circulation. 2012;**126**:349-356

[134] Sun XG, Hansen JE, Oudiz R, et al. Exercise pathophysiology in patients with primary pulmonary hypertension. Circulation. 2001;**104**:429-435

[135] Arena R, Lavie CJ, Milani RV, et al. Cardiopulmonary exercise testing in patients with pulmonary arterial hypertension: An evidence-based review. The Journal of Heart and Lung Transplantation. 2010;**29**:159-173

[136] Wensel R, Francis DP, Meyer FJ, et al. Incremental prognostic value of cardiopulmonary exercise testing and resting haemodynamics in pulmonary arterial hypertension. International Journal of Cardiology. 2013;**167**:1193-1198

[137] Raymond RJ, Hinderliter AL, Willis PW, et al. Echocardiographic predictors of adverse outcomes in primary pulmonary hypertension. Journal of the American College of Cardiology. 2002;**39**:1214-1219

[138] Bustamante-Labarta M, Perrone S, De La Fuente RL, et al. Right atrial size and tricuspid regurgitation severity predict mortality or transplantation in primary pulmonary hypertension. Journal of the American Society of Echocardiography. 2002;**15**:1160-1164

[139] Forfia PR, Fisher MR, Mathai SC, et al. Tricuspid annular displacement predicts survival in pulmonary

hypertension. American Journal of Respiratory and Critical Care Medicine. 2006;**174**:1034-1041

[140] Grunig E, Tiede H, Enyimayew EO, et al. Assessment and prognostic relevance of right ventricular contractile reserve in patients with severe pulmonary hypertension. Circulation. 2013;**128**:2005-2015

[141] Warwick G, Thomas PS, Yates DH. Biomarkers in pulmonary hypertension. The European Respiratory Journal. 2008;**32**:503-512

[142] Kumpers P, Nickel N, Lukasz A, et al. Circulating angiopoietins in idiopathic pulmonary arterial hypertension. European Heart Journal. 2010;**31**:2291-2300

[143] Quarck R, Nawrot T, Meyns B, et al. C-reactive protein: A new predictor of adverse outcome in pulmonary arterial hypertension. Journal of the American College of Cardiology. 2009;**53**:1211-1218

[144] Lorenzen JM, Nickel N, Kramer R, et al. Osteopontin in patients with idiopathic pulmonary hypertension. Chest. 2011;**139**:1010-1017

[145] Nagaya N, Nishikimi T, Uematsu M, et al. Plasma brain natriuretic peptide as a prognostic indicator in patients with primary pulmonary hypertension. Circulation. 2000;**102**:865-870

[146] Fijalkowska A, Kurzyna M, Torbicki A, et al. Serum N-terminal brain natriuretic peptide as a prognostic parameter in patients with pulmonary hypertension. Chest. 2006;**129**:1313-1321

[147] Williams MH, Handler C, Akram R, et al. Role of N-terminal brain natriuretic peptide (N-TproBNP) in scleroderma-associated pulmonary arterial hypertension. European Heart Journal. 2005;**27**:1485-1494

[148] Dimitroulas T, Giannakoulas G, Karvounis H, et al. Natriuretic peptides in systemic sclerosis-related pulmonary arterial hypertension. Seminars in Arthritis and Rheumatism. 2010;**39**:278-284

[149] Leuchte HH, El NM, Tuerpe JC, et al. N-terminal pro-brain natriuretic peptide and renal insufficiency as predictors of mortality in pulmonary hypertension. Chest. 2007;**131**:402-409

[150] Allanore Y, Borderie D, Meune C, et al. N-terminal pro-brain natriuretic peptide as a diagnostic marker of early pulmonary artery hypertension in patients with systemic sclerosis and effects of calcium channel blockers. Arthritis and Rheumatism. 2003;**48**:3503-3508

[151] Galie N, Ghofrani HA, Torbicki A, et al. Sildenafil citrate therapy for pulmonary arterial hypertension. The New England Journal of Medicine. 2005;**353**:2148-2157

[152] Badesch DB, Hill NS, Burgess G, et al. Sildenafil for pulmonary arterial hypertension associated with connective tissue disease. The Journal of Rheumatology. 2007;**34**:2417-2422

[153] Galie N, Brundage BH, Ghofrani HA, et al. Tadalafil therapy for pulmonary arterial hypertension. Circulation. 2009;**119**:2894-2903

[154] Jing ZC, Yu ZX, Shen JY, et al. Vardenafil in pulmonary arterial hypertension: A randomized, double-blind, placebo-controlled study. American Journal of Respiratory and Critical Care Medicine. 2011;**183**(12):1723-1729

[155] Ghofrani HA, Galie' N, Grimminger F, et al. Riociguat for the treatment of pulmonary arterial

hypertension. The New England Journal of Medicine. 2013;**369**:330-340

[156] Ghofrani HA, D'Armini AM, Grimminger F, et al. Riociguat for the treatment of chronic thromboembolic pulmonary hypertension. The New England Journal of Medicine. 2013;**369**:319-329

[157] Humbert M, Coghlan JG, Ghofrani HA, et al. Riociguat for the treatment of pulmonary arterial hypertension associated with connective tissue disease: results from PATENT-1 and PATENT-2. Annals of the Rheumatic Diseases. 2017;**76**:422-426

[158] Stewart DJ, Levy RD, Cernacek P, et al. Increased plasma endothelin-1 in pulmonary hypertension: Marker or mediator of disease? Annals of Internal Medicine. 1991;**114**:464-469

[159] Galie' N, Manes A, Branzi A. The endothelin system in pulmonary arterial hypertension. Cardiovascular Research. 2004;**61**:227-237

[160] Rubin LJ, Badesch DB, Barst RJ, et al. Bosentan therapy for pulmonary arterial hypertension. The New England Journal of Medicine. 2002;**346**:896-903

[161] Galie' N, Rubin LJ, Hoeper M, et al. Treatment of patients with mildly symptomatic pulmonary arterial hypertension with bosentan (EARLY study): A double-blind, randomized controlled trial. Lancet. 2008;**371**:2093-2100

[162] Galie' N, Beghetti M, Gatzoulis MA, et al. Bosentan therapy in patients with Eisenmenger syndrome: A multicenter, double-blind, randomized, placebo-controlled study. Circulation. 2006;**114**:48-54

[163] Channick RN, Simmoneau G, Sitbon O, et al. Effects of the dual endothelin receptor antagonist bosentan in patients with pulmonary hypertension: A randomized placebo-controlled study. Lancet. 2001;**358**:1119-1123

[164] Galie' N, Badesch BD, Oudiz R, et al. Ambrisentan therapy for pulmonary arterial hypertension. Journal of the American College of Cardiology. 2005;**46**:529-535

[165] Galie' N, Olschewski H, Oudiz R et al. Ambrisentan for the treatment of pulmonary arterial hypertension. Results of the ambrisentan in pulmonary arterial hypertension, randomized, double-blind, placebo-controlled, multicenter, efficacy (ARIES) study 1 and 2. Circulation 2008; 117: 3010-3019

[166] Pulido T, Adzerikho I, Channick RN, et al. Macitentan and morbidity and mortality in pulmonary arterial hypertension. The New England Journal of Medicine. 2013;**369**:809-818

[167] Galie' N, Manes A, Branzi A. Prostanoids for pulmonary arterial hypertension. American Journal of Respiratory Medicine. 2003;**2**:123-137

[168] Rubin LJ, Mendoza J, Hood M, et al. Treatment of primary pulmonary hypertension with continuous intravenous prostacyclin (epoprostenol). Results of a randomized trial. Annals of Internal Medicine. 1990;**112**:485-491

[169] Barst RJ, Rubin LJ, Long WA, et al. A comparison of continuous intravenous epoprostenol (prostacyclin) with conventional therapy for primary pulmonary hypertension. The New England Journal of Medicine. 1996;**334**:296-302

[170] Badesch DB, Tapson VF, McGoon MD, et al. Continuous intravenous epoprostenol for pulmonary hypertension due to the scleroderma spectrum of disease. A randomized, controlled trial. Annals of Internal Medicine. 2000;**132**:425-434

[171] Simmoneau G, Barst RJ, Galie' N, et al. Continuous subcutaneous infusion of treprostinil, a prostacyclin analogue, in patients with pulmonary arterial hypertension: A double-blind, randomized, placebo-controlled trial. American Journal of Respiratory and Critical Care Medicine. 2002;**165**:800-804

[172] Barst RJ, Galie' N, Naeije R, et al. Long-term outcome in pulmonary arterial hypertension patients treated with subcutaneous treprostinil. The European Respiratory Journal. 2006;**28**:1195-1203

[173] McLaughlin V, Rubin L, Benza RL, et al. Addition of inhaled treprostinil to oral therapy for pulmonary arterial hypertension: A randomized controlled clinical trial. Journal of the American College of Cardiology. 2010;**55**:1915-1922

[174] Jing ZC, Parikh K, Pulido T, et al. Efficacy and safety of oral treprostinil monotherapy for the treatment of pulmonary arterial hypertension: A randomized, controlled trial. Circulation. 2013;**127**:624-633

[175] Olschewski H, Simmoneau G, Galie' N, et al. Inhaled iloprost in severe pulmonary hypertension. The New England Journal of Medicine. 2002;**347**:322-329

[176] Higenbottam T, Butt AY, McMahon A, et al. Long-term intravenous prostaglandin (epoprostenol or iloprost) for treatment of severe pulmonary hypertension. Heart. 1998;**80**:151-155

[177] Norel X. Prostanoid receptors in the human vascular wall. Scientific World Journal. 2007;**7**:1359-1374

[178] Humbert M, Lau EM, Montani D, et al. Advances in therapeutic interventions for patients with pulmonary arterial hypertension. Circulation. 2014;**130**:2189-2208

[179] Mubarak KK. A review of prostaglandin analogues in the management of patients with pulmonary arterial hypertension. Respiratory Medicine. 2010;**104**:9-21

[180] McLaughlin VV, Channick R, Chin KM, et al. Effect of selexipag on morbidity/mortality in pulmonary arterial hypertension: Results of the GRIPHON study. Journal of the American College of Cardiology. 2015;**65**(Suppl A):A380

[181] Sitbon O, Channick R, Chin KM, et al. Selexipag for the treatment of pulmonary arterial hypertension. The New England Journal of Medicine. 2015;**373**:2522-2533

[182] Gaine S, Chin K, Coghlan G, et al. Selexipag for the treatment of connective tissue disease-associated pulmonary arterial hypertension. The European Respiratory Journal. 2017;**50**:1602493

[183] Galie N, Barbara JA, Frost A, et al. Initial use of ambrisentan plus tadalafil in pulmonary arterial hypertension. New England Journal of Medicine. 2015;**379**:834-844

[184] Coghlan JG, Galie' N, Barbera JA, et al. Initial combination therapy with ambrisentan and tadalafil in connective tissue disease-associated pulmonary arterial hypertension (CTD-PAH): Subgroup analysis from the AMBITION trial. Annals of the Rheumatic Diseases. 2017;**76**:1219-1227

[185] Hassoun PM, Zamanian RT, Damico R, et al. Ambrisentan and tadalafil up-front combination therapy in scleroderma-associated pulmonary arterial hypertension. American Journal of Respiratory and Critical Care Medicine. 2015;**192**:1102-1110

[186] Taichman DB, Ornelas J, Chung L, et al. Pharmacologic therapy for pulmonary arterial hypertension in

adults. CHEST guideline and expert panel report. Chest. 2014;**146**:449-475

[187] Kurzyna M, Dabrowski M, Bielecki D, et al. Atrial septostomy in treatment of end-stage right heart failure in patients with pulmonary hypertension. Chest. 2007;**131**:977-983

[188] Sandoval J, Gaspar J, Pulido T, et al. Graded balloon dilation atrial septostomy in severe primary pulmonary hypertension. A therapeutic alternative for patients nonresponsive to vasodilator treatment. Journal of the American College of Cardiology. 1998;**32**:297-304

[189] Khan IY, Singer LG, de Perrot M, et al. Survival after lung transplantation in systemic sclerosis. A systematic review. Respiratory Medicine. 2013;**107**:2081-2087

[190] deMendonca L, Felix ND, Blanco NG, et al. Mesenchymal stromal cell therapy reduces lung inflammation and vascular remodeling and improves hemodynamics in experimental pulmonary arterial hypertension. Stem Cell Research and Therapy. 2017;**8**:220

[191] Mereles D, Ehlken N, Kreuscher S, et al. Exercise and respiratory training improve exercise capacity and quality of life in patients with severe chronic pulmonary hypertension. Circulation. 2006;**114**:1482-1489

[192] Grunig E, Maier F, Ehlken N, et al. Exercise training in pulmonary arterial hypertension associated with connective tissue diseases. Arthritis Research and Therapy. 2012;**14**:R148

[193] Bonnin M, Mercier FJ, Sitbon O, et al. Severe pulmonary hypertension during pregnancy: mode of delivery and anesthetic management of 15 consecutive cases. Anesthesiology. 2005;**102**:1133-1137

[194] Guillevin L, Armstrong I, Aldrighetti R, et al. Understanding the impact of pulmonary arterial hypertension on patients' and carers' lives. European Respiratory Review. 2013;**22**:535-542

[195] Soubrier F, Chung WK, Machado R, et al. Genetics and genomics of pulmonary arterial hypertension. Journal of the American College of Cardiology. 2013;**62**(Suppl):D13-D21

[196] Ramakrishnan G, Sprung J, Ravi BS, et al. Impact of pulmonary hypertension on the outcomes of noncardiac surgery: Predictors of perioperative mobidity and mortality. Journal of the American College of Cardiology. 2005;**45**:1691-1699

[197] McGlothlin D, DeMarco T. Preoperative risk assessment of pulmonary arterial hypertension. Patients undergoing general surgery. Advances in Pulmonary Arterial Hypertension. 2007;**6**(2):66-73

[198] Minai OA, Yared JP, Kaw R, et al. Perioperative risk and management in patients with pulmonary hypertension. Chest. 2013;**144**:329-340

[199] Meyer S, McLaughlin VV, Seyfarth HJ, et al. Outcomes of noncardiac, nonobstetric surgery in patients with PAH: An international prospective survey. The European Respiratory Journal. 2013;**41**:1302-1307

Chapter 2

Renal Involvement in Systemic Sclerosis

Tomas Soukup, Jan Toms, Sabina Oreska, Eva Honsova and Roman Safranek

Abstract

Scleroderma renal crisis (SRC) is classical renal disease in systemic sclerosis (SSc). SRC is a relatively rare manifestation, approximately in 5% of patients. In terms of severity, manifestation in the form of SRC is the most common cause of acute organ failure. In SSc patients, SRC is defined as a new onset of accelerated arterial hypertension and rapidly progressive anuric or oliguric renal failure. SRC is primarily vascular injury with increased activity of the renin-angiotensin activity. These events lead to release or activation of cytokines and growth factors that result in the typical proliferative vascular lesions. Successful approach is routine use of angiotensin-converting enzyme inhibitors in the treatment of SRC (except prevention) and other advances in renal replacement therapy in SSc management. It is crucial to detect manifestations of SRC early and to manage appropriately in collaboration with intensive care medicine, cardiologists, and nephrologists. In contrast to SRC, clinical presentation of interstitial renal disease is poor, often without evidence of renal abnormality. Interestingly, other renal manifestations are glomerulonephritis and vasculitis. These manifestations are associated with overlapping mechanisms. The objective of this chapter is to focus on actual knowledge about the renal involvement in SSc and current treatment principles and possibilities.

Keywords: kidney, systemic sclerosis, scleroderma renal crisis, glomerulonephritis, diagnosis, management

1. Introduction

Systemic sclerosis (SSc) leads to morbidity and mortality through a combination of inflammation, fibrosis, and vascular damage leading to internal organ complications affecting the heart, lung, bowel, and kidneys. In SSc, we observe kidney involvement as three main clinical situations described below.

Most often, SSc causes a range of renal manifestations, which occur in both subsets of the disease: limited cutaneous (lcSSc) and diffuse cutaneous (dcSSc) subsets.

As overlaps are often seen in connective tissue diseases, SSc should be associated with other immunological features of renal disease findings typical for systemic lupus erythematosus (as lupus glomerulonephritis) and ANCA-associated vasculitis/glomerulonephritis.

Scleroderma renal crisis (SRC) is a dramatic and classical scleroderma manifestation, historically known as dominant cause of scleroderma-related death. Currently, the leading causes of death in scleroderma are pulmonary fibrosis and pulmonary arterial hypertension [1]. Regardless, one-year SRC outcomes remain poor, with over 30% mortality and 25% of patients remaining dialysis-dependent.

To make the summary complete, possible drug-related adverse events including from toxic renal involvement to renal acute renal failure must be mentioned.

2. Scleroderma renal crisis

2.1 Epidemiology

SRC occurs usually in early dcSSc (11%), as compared to patients with lcSSc (4%) [2, 3]. SRC is more common in rapidly progressing disease, SRC was previously reported up to 25% of SSc, but over time, it was found that incidence of renal crisis appeared to have decreased since improvement of early diagnostics [1].

Historically, study of Steen and Medsger [4] presented change of mortality causes during 1972–2002 years. This study showed that SRC as the cause decreased from 42 to 6% of SSc-related deaths, while the proportion of other causes of death increased: pulmonary fibrosis rose from 6 to 33% and pulmonary arterial hypertension from 22 to 28%. Large data were obtained prospectively followed in the EULAR Scleroderma Trials and Research (EUSTAR) cohort. The EUSTAR database was inaugurated in June 2004 and represents a multinational, prospective, and open SSc cohort [5]. According to EUSTAR data, SSc-related deaths include pulmonary fibrosis 19%, pulmonary arterial hypertension 14%, arrhythmia 6%, heart failure 7%, and SRC 4%. Non–SSc-related deaths in total 4% include infection 13%, malignancy 13%, and cardiovascular 12%. Renal causes accounted for the death of 10 patients (4%), all due to renal crisis. Renal crisis was fatal in 16% of all patients experiencing renal crisis [5].

2.2 Pathogenesis of scleroderma renal crisis

Pathogenesis is characterized by series of insults (**Figure 1**):

- *Changes in intima and endothelium*: Initially, there is injury to the endothelial cells with intimal thickening and proliferation in the arcuate and interlobular arteries [6].

- *Absence of inflammation*: There is a notable absence of inflammatory cells (lymphocytes and monocytes) in the renal vasculature [6].

- *Vascular injury*: Platelet factors are released causing increased vascular permeability, fibrin deposition, and collagen formation, which lead to further luminal narrowing [6].

- *Renal ischemia*: Narrowed renal arterioles decrease renal cortical blood flow [6].

- *Activation of renin*: Renal ischemia and episodic renal vasospasm "renal Raynaud phenomenon" contribute to decrease of blood flow. Decreased renal blood flow causes hyperplasia of the juxtaglomerular apparatus and release of renin [6].

- *Secondary small vessel changes*: endothelial injury is associated with thrombus formation. Intravascular thrombi and mucoid intimal edema may be seen in renal histology. Small vessel thrombi are more abundant than glomerular

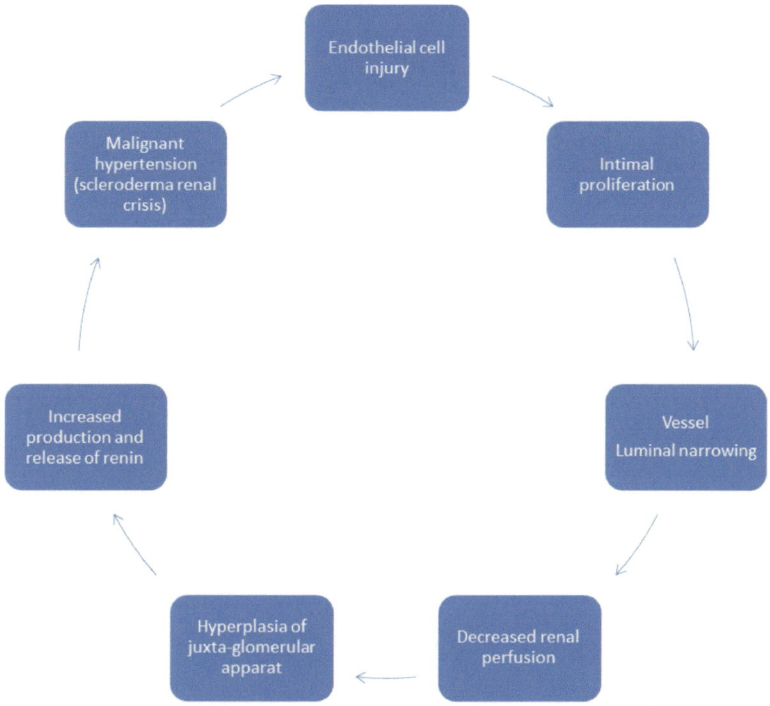

Figure 1.
The mechanisms in the pathogenesis of SRC. Adapted from Steen et al. [8].

thrombi (unlike the pathology seen in hemolytic-uremic syndrome and thrombotic thrombocytopenic purpura) [7].

2.3 Renal histopathology

Histopathological findings of SRC are more frequently manifested by severe involvement of small arteries and arterioles. Early vascular changes are characterized by intimal accumulation of myxoid material in the interlobular and arcuate arteries, which results in severe luminal narrowing (**Figure 2**). Sometimes microthrombi are developed in the affected vessels and fragmented red blood cells can be

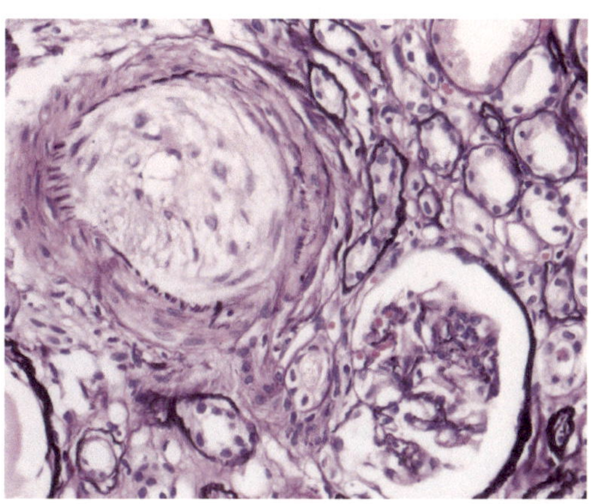

Figure 2.
Early vascular changes are characterized by intimal accumulation of pale myxoid material in the small artery, which results in severe luminal narrowing (Methenamine-silver stain).

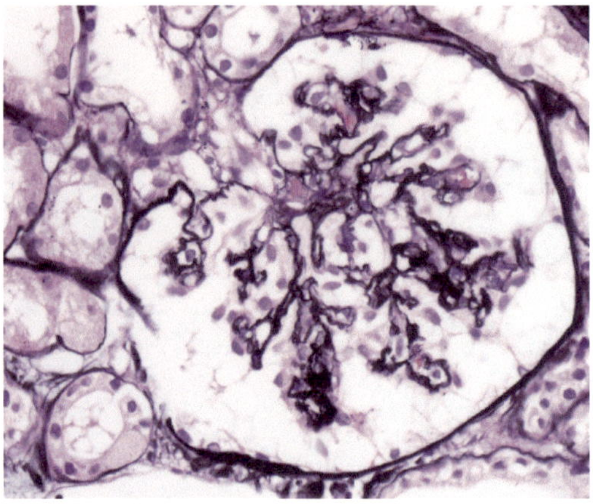

Figure 3.
Two types of glomerular injury associated with scleroderma renal crisis. Ischemic collapse of glomerulus with wrinkling of glomerular basement membrane corresponds to arterial stenosis.

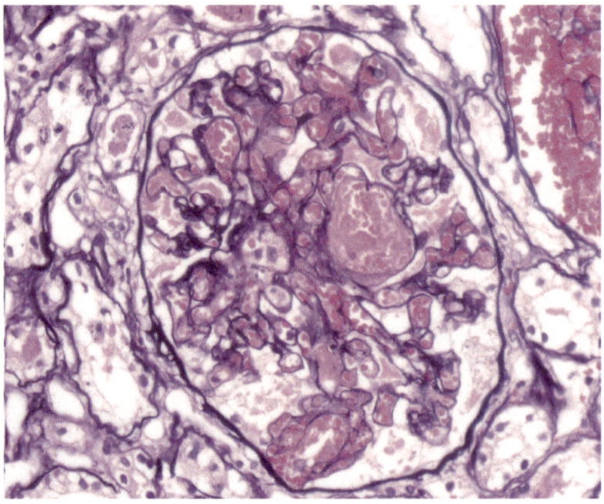

Figure 4.
Two types of glomerular injury associated with scleroderma renal crisis. Thrombotic microangiopathy with occlusion of outgoing arteriole is characterized by the congestion and hemorrhagic necrosis of the tuft (Methenamine-silver stain).

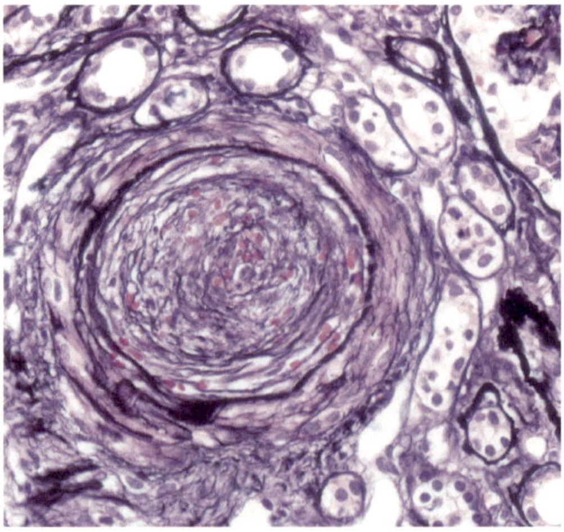

Figure 5.
Prominent intimal concentric lamination within an interlobular artery (arterial onion skin lesion) with irreversible reduction of the arterial lumen (Methenamine-silver stain).

seen in vessel wall. Microthrombi in arterioles can also progress to the glomeruli. When the arterioles incoming to glomeruli are predominantly affected, the morphological features in glomeruli are characterized by ischemia with wrinkling of glomerular basement membrane and ischemic collapses of glomeruli (**Figure 3**). When microthrombi are developed mainly in outgoing arterioles, the corresponding pathology is severe congestion and hemorrhagic necrosis of the tufts (**Figure 4**).

Later arterial injury is characterized by change of edematous mucoid intima to the concentric lamination and so called onion skin lesion (**Figure 5**) with significant luminal reduction. In glomeruli, the lesion is represented by double contouring of glomerular basement membrane (as a result of prolonged or repeated endothelial injury) and segmental or global sclerotic lesions.

Because blood supply in the kidney is represented by end vessels without collaterals, each area of kidney tissue after arterial luminal narrowing must suffer from severe ischemia or even tissue necrosis. In histopathology, pronounced ischemia leads to tubular injury in the intersticium and tubular atrophy with interstitial fibrosis in the course of time.

Since none of these findings are specific for SRC, the pathological diagnosis must be supported by appropriate clinical and serological data [9].

Histopathology: with courtesy of Eva Honsová, MD., PhD. Department of Pathology IKEM, Prague.

2.4 Definition, diagnosis, and classification

SRC is defined as new onset of accelerated arterial hypertension and rapidly progressive oliguric renal failure during the course of SSc. There are differences between the criteria used to *define SRC* [1]. Occasionally, more modest elevations in blood pressure and renal dysfunction and at times normotensive presentations were found [9, 10]. The diagnosis is complicated in the case of malignant hypertension with absence of kidney impairment.

SRC was defined in a minority of studies and criteria were heterogeneous [10]. It is a problem to establish criteria for SRC, because the clinical spectrum of SRC is broad, ranging from accelerated hypertension to normotensive patients 7% [10]. Arterial hypertension is a typical symptom in SRC accompanied by classical complications such as hypertensive encephalopathy, retinopathy, congestive heart failure, hemolysis, etc. Diagnosis of SRC in patients without pre-existing SSc diagnosis and in normotensive SRC patients is difficult, mainly in the absence of renal biopsy [10, 11].

Only one study up to now has partially validated criteria for SRC (**Table 1**) [8]. It was proposed by experts in 2003. It included items for systolic and diastolic blood pressure, serum creatinine, proteinuria, hematuria, microangiopathic hemolytic anemia, and renal histopathology. These are known as the Ancona criteria for SRC [8].

Recently, the Scleroderma Clinical Trials Consortium (SCTC) and Scleroderma Renal Crisis Working Group generate a core set of items to develop classification criteria for SRC using Delphi methodology. The final core set of items to develop classification criteria for SRC contains domains: blood pressure arise, kidney impairment, hematological changes, thrombotic microangiopathy, and organ dysfunction. A consensus definition of SRC is urgently needed to standardize data collection on SRC [9].

Novel concepts of SRC classification included the stratification of SRC:

- *definite SRC*: defined as at least two of: new onset hypertension, microangiopathic hemolytic anemia (MAHA), and rising creatinine

- *subacute forms of SRC*: such as hypertension, renal insufficiency, and renal sediment changes in the absence of microangiopathic hemolytic anemia [9, 10]

SRC is defined as following, requiring both:

A new onset of blood pressure >150/85 mm Hg obtained at least twice over a consecutive 24-hour period. This blood pressure is chosen because it is defined by the New York Heart Association as significant hypertension.

Decrease in the renal function as defined by a decrement of at least 10% in the estimated GFR (eGFR) or GFR of <90 (mL/min/1.73 m^2. When possible, a repeat serum creatinine and recalculation of the GFR should be obtained to corroborate the initial results.

In order to corroborate further the occurrence of acute renal crisis, it would be desirable to have any of the following, if available:

- new onset of urinary red blood cells (excluding other causes)
- flash pulmonary edema
- oliguria or anuria
- microangiopathic hemolytic anemia on blood smear
- retinopathy typical of acute hypertensive crisis
- renal biopsy with typical features including onion skin proliferation within the walls of internal arteries and arterioles, fibrinoid necrosis, and glomerular shrinkage

Notes

- Cases of typical SRC histological appearance have been associated with scleroderma in the absence of hypertension; these cases of normotensive SRC are reported to have a particularly poor outcome, and their precise relationship to the more typical hypertensive SRC is not known. Normotensive SRC was observed in glucocorticoid scleroderma users.
- Up to one fifth of cases of SRC with hypertension have been identified as the presenting feature of systemic sclerosis, and so, in these cases, pre-existing diagnosis of systemic sclerosis will not be present.

SRC, scleroderma renal crisis; GFR, glomerular filtration rate.

Table 1.
Clinical criteria for definition of scleroderma renal crisis [1].

New concept also includes the addition of ACE inhibitor responsiveness as a characteristic of hypertension (in *probable SRC*) and the addition of more specific time frames for measurement of blood pressure (taken twice, 2 hours apart, within 3 days of first event-associated observation) [10].

In addition to heterogeneity and rarity, the absence of a gold standard and classification criteria are important challenges for research on SRC. The development of new criteria is important to improve the definition of normotensive SRC. In this case, performing kidney biopsy and examination of biomarkers (including anti-RNA III polymerase) are important and promising.

2.5 Role of kidney biopsy in diagnosis of scleroderma renal crisis

Kidney biopsy is not mandatory for diagnosis of SRC. In patients at risk of SRC with its typical clinical presentation, kidney biopsy is usually not performed. However, it should be considered in all patients with atypical presentation and findings, especially in normotensive patients, patients with ANCA positivity, severe proteinuria, and nephrotic syndrome.

In most patients, we cannot perform kidney biopsy immediately as severe hypertension and frequently present thrombocytopenia significantly increase the risk of bleeding. Biopsy is usually performed within a few days after blood pressure correction and is done with reasonably low risk in patients with blood pressure below 160/90 mmHg and thrombocyte count above 100×10^9/l.

2.6 Predictive and risk factors

Identification of SRC predictive factors (before the development of SRC) is essential (**Table 2**). The vast majority of SRC cases (75–80%) occur in patients with diffuse skin involvement, i.e., skin scleroderma proximal to knee and elbow (dcSSc patients), and rapid progression of skin thickening has been shown to be associated with the development of SRC [12]. Arthritis, palpable tendon friction rubs, swollen fingers, and distal parts of hands are routine syndrome in patients with early dcSSc [13]. Tendon friction rubs were confirmed to be an independent predictor of SRC (HR: 2.33) [14].

SRC starts early, most often less than 4 years after the first SSc symptom, although SRC patients have minimal or even no skin changes at the time of the diagnosis of SRC. Males are proportionately more frequently affected than females [15].

On the other hand, patients previously called as CREST (calcinosis, Raynaud phenomenon, esophageal dysmotility, sclerodactyly and Telangiectasia) rarely develop SRC. These patients are subgroup of lcSSc fundamentally [12].

When talking about risk factors of death, a history of renal crisis (HR 2.89), presence of proteinuria (HR 3.09), elevated acute phase reactants (HR 1.79), elevated creatine kinase (HR 1.73), and muscle weakness (HR 1.55) were associated with decreased survival [5, 16]. On the other hand, since the introduction of ACE inhibitors, renal crisis appears to have become an increasingly less frequent terminal event [4]. In EUSTAR cohort, except one individual, all patients dying from renal crisis were on an ACE inhibitor at the time of death. Prednisone equivalents above 15 mg daily have been implicated in exacerbating SRC [5].

Several retrospective studies suggest that glucocorticoids are associated with a higher risk of SRC. Blood pressure and renal function should be carefully monitored in patients with SSc treated with glucocorticoids [17]. Evidence regarding the impact of steroid use on the development of SRC comes mainly from retrospective studies, most of which showed significant association between steroid exposure and the occurrence of SRC [11, 15, 18–22].

A retrospective analysis including 140 patients with SRC showed that high doses of steroids (prednisone ≥30 mg/day) were used frequently in patients with SSc with normotensive SRC (64%) as compared with those with hypertensive SRC (16%) suggesting an association between the use of high-dose steroids and the risk of normotensive SRC, which is associated with worse prognosis [11].

Glucocorticoids are routinely used for the management of interstitial lung disease, puffy fingers, and skin involvement. These indications are not recommended (because of insufficient evidence of efficacy); however, the experts recognize their use in everyday practice in the management of inflammatory manifestations such as musculoskeletal involvement (arthritis, tendonitis, myositis—in overlap with idiopathic inflammatory myopaties), pericarditis, pleuritis (in overlap with SLE), nonspecific symptoms such as skin itching/burning, fatigue, and appetite (with empiric basis) [17, 23]. Considering the potential risk of SRC associated with steroid use, the experts recommend that patients with SSc treated with steroids should be carefully monitored with respect to the development of SRC [17].

It can be summarized that glucocorticoids have a very narrow or no therapeutic opportunity in SSc.

SRC patient-specific characteristics
Race—black
Gender—male sex
SSc characteristics
Short course of SSc
Diffuse cutaneous systemic scleroderma
Modified Rodnan skin score (>14 or 20)
Musculoskeletal contractures
Tendon friction rubs
Pitting scars on finger tips
Cardiopulmonary manifestation
Heart failure
Pericarditis
FVC <75% expected value
DLCO low/decrease
Muscle involvement
Muscle weakness
Higher creatine kinase level
Myalgias or myopathy
Arthritis/Arthralgias
Genetics and biomarkers
Anti-RNA polymerase III presence
Anti-RNA polymerase I/II/III presence
ELISA anti-RNA polymerase III ≥157 IU
Anti-centromere absence
Anti-nRNP presence
ANA speckled immunofluorescence
lipocalin-2 high levels [24]
sCD147 high levels [25]
angiogenin high levels
endothelin-1 high levels
HLA-DRB1*0407
HLA-DRB1*1304
Risk factors developed during SSc
Skin changes acceleration
Hemoglobin, thrombocyte decrease
Cardiac involvement—new
Pericarditis
Congestive heart failure
Drugs
Cocaine [26]
Glucocorticoid treatment
Cyclosporine A
Absence of calcium channel blocker
Factors without evidence of SRC risk
Previous blood pressure arise
Abnormal dip-stick and light proteinuria
Chronic elevation of serum creatinine
Presence of antibodies: anti-topoisomerase, anti-centromere

SRC, scleroderma renal crisis; SSc, systemic sclerosis; FVC, forced lung vital capacity; DLCO, diffusing capacity for carbon monoxide; RNA, ribonucleic acid; ELISA, enzyme-linked immunosorbent assay; nRNP, nucleic ribonucleic protein; ANA, antinuclear antibodies; HLA, human leucocyte antigen.

Table 2.
Clinical and laboratory predictors of scleroderma renal crisis and worse outcome. Adapted from Bose et al. [6].

2.7 Clinical manifestation of scleroderma renal crisis

2.7.1 Early symptoms

Sometimes SRC symptoms are nonspecific, for example, fatigue or not feeling well. Typically, patients complain of severe headache, blurred vision, or other encephalopathic symptoms with the onset of accelerated hypertension. Seizures may be also an early finding [1].

2.7.2 Blood pressure

Most patients have striking increase of blood pressure at the onset of SRC. Above 90% patients have blood pressure levels >150/90 mm Hg, 30% have diastolic pressure >120 mm Hg, and <10% of SSc have a normal blood pressure. In addition to thinking about absolute values, clinically important risk factors arise of 30 mmHg systolic and 20 mmHg diastolic blood pressure (repeatedly measured) [1].

2.7.3 Kidney injury, conditio sine qua non

Acute kidney injury is defined as any of the following: increase in serum creatinine by >26.5 μmol/L (> 0.3 mg/dl) within 48 hours; increase in serum creatinine to >1.5 times baseline, which is known or presumed to have occurred within the prior 7 days, and urine volume <0.5 ml/kg/h for 6 hours. This is the definition of acute kidney injury from the Kidney Disease Improving Global Outcomes (KDIGO) guidelines [27].

2.7.4 Cardiopulmonary system

Patients with SRC often present with congestive heart failure presented as dyspnea, paroxysmal nocturnal dyspnea or pulmonary edema, serious ventricular arrhythmias, cardiac arrest, or large pericardial effusion [11]. Interestingly, this is primarily owing to the stress of hypertension on the heart, effects of hyperreninemia, and fluid overload secondary to oliguric renal failure. Some patients have primary scleroderma myocardial involvement contributing to these consecutive insults [1].

Acute pericarditis is diagnosed if the patient has at least 2 of the 4 following criteria: (1) pericarditis chest pain; (2) pericardial rub; (3) new widespread ST-elevation or PR depression on electrocardiogram; (4) pericardial effusion (new or worsening) on cardiac echocardiography [1].

Pulmonary hemorrhage is a rare life-threatening status, which has occurred in several of SRC patients [10]. Etiopathogenesis is associated with pulmonary edema and hemorrhagic diathesis. In differential diagnosis, diffuse alveolar hemorrhagia and acute renal failure were rarely observed in cases of ANCA systemic vasculitis and SSc overlaps [28].

2.7.5 Target organ dysfunction

Typically, hypertensive retinopathy (hemorrhages, hard and soft (cotton wool) exudates, and/or disc edema, not attributable to other causes), confirmed by an ophthalmologist, is observed. Hypertensive encephalopathy is characterized by headache, altered mental status, seizures, visual disturbances, and/or other focal or diffuse neurologic signs not attributable to other causes. Acute congestive heart failure is characterized by typical symptoms (e.g., breathlessness, ankle swelling, and fatigue) that may be accompanied by signs (e.g., elevated jugular venous pressure, pulmonary crackles, and peripheral edema) [1, 6].

2.8 Laboratory findings

2.8.1 Autoantibodies

Antinuclear antibodies (ANA) are hallmark of connective tissue diseases. In case of Raynaud phenomenon, puffy fingers, nailfold capillaroscopy finding with typical microvascular changes, and ANA can alert to the very early diagnosis of SSc and may determine etiology of malignant hypertension. ANA are seen in 95% of SSc.

The presence of scleroderma-specific antibodies may confirm SSc diagnosis, anti-topoisomerase I predicts diffuse SSc, but only 10% of SRC has anti-topoisomerase I positivity [6, 29] (**Figure 6**).

Anti-RNA polymerase III is a scleroderma-specific antibody and is seen only in diffuse scleroderma. About 24–33% of these patients develop SRC [30–32]. It was showed that anti-RNA polymerase is strongly associated with SRC, OR 6.4 [33]. This statement is valid with the exception of geographical variability. For example, the difference in prevalence of autoantibodies among SRC patients between the Italian and other population might originate from the lower prevalence of anti-RNA polymerase III among Italians [34]. Anti-RNA polymerase III is associated with worse prognosis of SRC including Dialysis, persistence on dialysis, and survival [1].

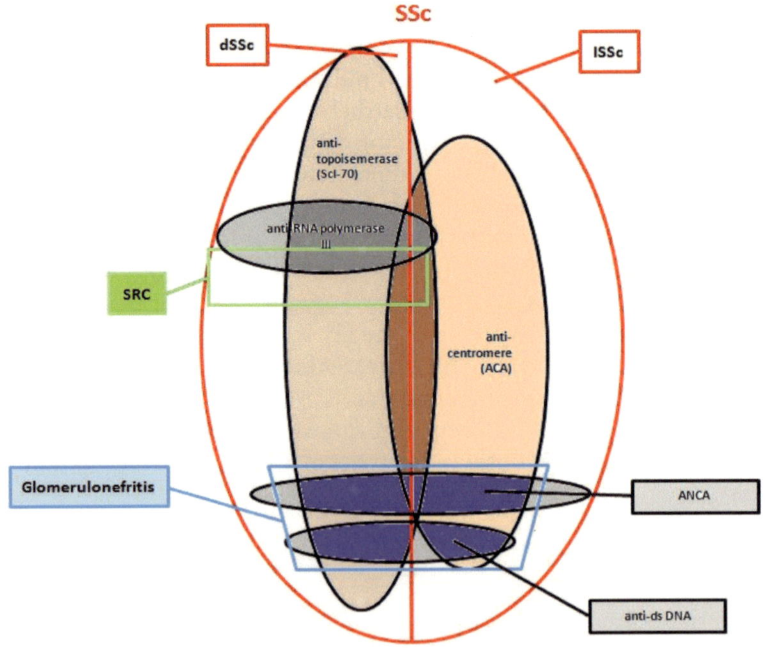

Figure 6.
Diagram showing subsets of systemic sclerosis associated with kidney involvement stratified by antibodies. Colored areas represent approximated proportion in patients. Adapted from Kuwana M and Medsger A [35]. SSc, systemic sclerosis; SRC, dSSc, diffuse cutaneous systemic sclerosis; lSSc, limited cutaneous systemic sclerosis; scleroderma renal crisis; anti-RNA polymerase III, anti-ribonucleic acid polymerase III antibodies; ANCA, anti-neutrophil cytoplasmic antibodies; anti-ds DNA, antibodies against double-stranded (ds) DNA.

2.8.2 Microangiopathic hemolytic anemia and thrombocytopenia

SRC is a disease characterized by thrombotic microangiopathy with typical blood laboratory findings—new or worsening anemia, presence of schistocytes or other red blood cell fragments in peripheral blood smear, and thrombocytopenia <100.000, confirmed by manual smear. Typical features are laboratory evidence of hemolysis, including elevated lactate dehydrogenase, reticulocytosis, and/or low/absent haptoglobin and negative direct anti-globulin test. In differential diagnosis, other types of thrombotic microangiopathies need to be excluded (see **Table 3**). In some cases, thrombotic thrombocytopenic purpura has been reported in scleroderma patients, but it is unclear whether it was an isolated coexisting disease or a different interpretation of SRC [1, 6, 36].

2.9 Differential diagnosis of scleroderma renal crisis

The most common differential diagnoses are

- anti-neutrophil cytoplasmic antibody (ANCA)-associated glomerulonephritis,
- lupus nephritis, and
- diseases associated with thrombotic microangiopathy (**Table 4**).

Thrombotic thrombocytopenic purpura (TTP) /hemolytic-uremic syndrome (HUS)/disseminated intravascular coagulation (DIC)/heparin-induced thrombocytopenia (HIT)/ pre-eclampsia or HELLP syndrome refers to an acronym used to describe the clinical condition that leads to hemolysis, elevated liver enzymes, and low platelets/catastrophic antiphospholipid syndrome (CAPS), etc. [37].

Other differential diagnoses reported included membranous and membranoproliferative nephropathies, other vasculitis (including polyarteritis nodosa, mixed cryoglobulinemia, and Goodpasture syndrome), drug-induced nephropathies (due to D-penicillamine or cyclosporin A), oxalate nephropathy, renal artery stenosis, and pre-renal causes (e.g., sepsis and dehydration) [10].

2.10 Management of scleroderma renal crisis

2.10.1 Prevention

Despite significant decrease in incidence of SRC, no reliable preventive measures were identified. To decrease the risk of SRC development, we have to identify patients at high risk. Risk factors are discussed above (see chapter "Predictive and Risk Factors"), and we should take special caution in patients with dSS in the early stages of the disease (less than 5 years from diagnosis) with rapid progression of skin thickening, palpable tendon friction rubs, and anti-RNAP III antibodies [39]. Clinically, most important modifiable factor seems to be glucocorticoid treatment. Doses as high as 15 mg of prednisone are associated with increased incidence of SRC in several studies (see below).

Patients at risk should have their blood pressure controlled well. However, ACE inhibitors that are recommended for SRC treatment have not been shown to have protective effect before SRC onset and do not improve outcome of SRC [18, 19]. On the other hand, there are some reports of negative impact of ACE inhibitors on worse outcome of SRC, if ACE inhibitors were used in prevention of SRC [1, 40].

History and condition	Scleroderma renal crisis	CAPS	TTP-HUS	HELLP syndrome	Sepsis	DIC	HIT
Previous history	Systemic sclerosis	APS/SLE/malignancy/ pregnancy	Malignancy/ non	pregnancy	infection	Infection/ malignancy	Heparin exposure
Thrombosis	Small vessels	Large/small vessels	Small vessels	Small vessels	Large/small vessels	Small vessels	Large/small vessels
Hemolytic anemia	+	−/+	++	+	−/+	−/+	—
Schistocytes	+	−/+	++	+	−/+	−/+	—
Fibrinogen	Normal/high	Normal/high	Normal/high	Normal/high	Normal/low	Normal/low	Normal/high
Typical antibodies	anti-RNA polymerase III	aPL	ADAMTS13	None	None	None	Anti-PF-4

TTP, thrombotic thrombocytopenic purpura; HUS, hemolytic uremic syndrome; DIC, disseminated intravascular coagulation; HELLP, hemolysis, elevated liver enzymes and low platelets syndrome; HIT, heparin-induced thrombocytopenia; APS, antiphospholipid syndrome; CAPS, catastrophic antiphospholipid syndrome; SLE, systemic lupus erythematosus; aPL, antiphospholipid antibodies; ADAMTS13, a disintegrin and metalloproteinase with a thrombospondin type 1 motif, member 13; PF-4, platelet factor 4.

Table 3.
Differential diagnosis of thrombotic microangiopathies from the view of scleroderma renal crisis. Adapted from Cervera et al. [37].

Event	Differences from SRC
Essential hypertension	Without acute renal failure
ANCA-associated glomerulonephritis	ANCA positivity, significant Proteinuria, hematuria [38]
Overlaps with connective tissue disease with glomerulonephritis (SLE)	Anti-dsDNA positivity, other CTD-specific antibodies
Renal artery stenosis	Absence of systemic symptoms
Thrombotic microangiopathies	
Pre-eclampsia	*Pregnancy*
Hemolytic uremic syndrome	*Shigella toxin*
Thrombocytic thrombocytopenic purpura	*ADAMTS13 antibody*
Catastrophic antiphospholipid syndrome	*Antiphospholipid antibodies*
Heparin-induced thrombocytopenia	*Heparin treatment*

Other conditions: membranous nephropathy, drug-induced nephropathies (e.g., cyclosporin A), other vasculitis (e.g., polyarteritis nodosa, mixed cryoglobulinemia, and Goodpasture syndrome), oxalate nephropathy, membranoproliferative nephropathy, pre-renal causes (e.g., sepsis, dehydration, and cardiac or pulmonary vascular involvement), and isolated renal abnormalities. SRC, scleroderma renal crisis; ANCA, antibodies against neutrophils; SLE, systemic lupus erythematosus; CTD, connective tissue diseases; ADAMTS13, a disintegrin and metalloproteinase with a thrombospondin type 1 motif, member 13.

Table 4.
Differential diagnosis of scleroderma renal crisis. Adapted from Bose et al. [6].

Therefore, other antihypertensive drugs should be used to treat primary hypertension in these patients. Calcium channel blockers are a preferred option, as these drugs are effective in controlling blood pressure and a positive vasodilatory effect [41].

2.10.2 Early diagnosis

Early diagnosis and treatment can significantly improve prognosis of the patients. Patients at risk should be instructed to monitor blood pressure at home at least twice a week. They should report sudden increase in blood pressure and blood pressure above 140/90 mmHg. These patients should have their blood pressure quickly normalized and should be evaluated for possible SRC development (evaluation of kidney function, presence of MAHA, etc.).

2.10.3 Treatment of scleroderma renal crisis

Current treatment of SSc focuses on broad-spectrum immunosuppression or organ-based therapy for separate manifestations such as lung fibrosis, skin and gastrointestinal involvement, pulmonary or systemic hypertension, and kidney impairment [1]. The treatment of SRC is based on three main principles: causal treatment with ACE inhibitors, methods of renal function replacement, and plasma exchange in some patients. For organ complications, supportive treatment is used. SRC without treatment is often lethal. SRC patients should be treated immediately and aggressively with hospitalization and under careful control (**Figure** 7) [1]. It is advisable to admit patients with symptomatic hypertension to intensive care units.

2.10.3.1 Angiotensin-converting enzyme inhibitors

The key to improved outcome is treatment with ACE inhibitors. It should be initiated as soon as possible. Captopril is the preferred option. It has been used in

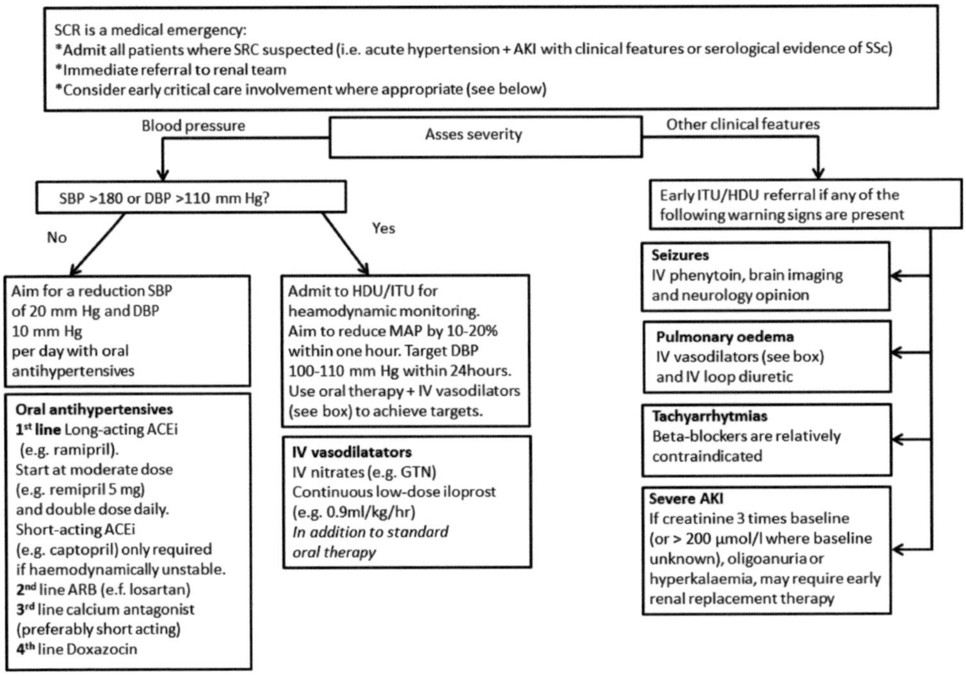

Figure 7.
Management of scleroderma renal crisis, adapted from Lynch et al. [50]. ACEi, angiotensin-converting enzyme inhibitor; AKI, acute kidney injury; ARB, angiotensin receptor blocker; DBP, diastolic blood pressure; HDU, high dependency unit; ITU, intensive therapy unit; MAP, mean arterial pressure; SBP, systolic blood pressure.

most studies and its short-acting character enables good titration at the start of the treatment. It is usually necessary to use very high doses. Blood pressure should be brought back to normal levels within 2–4 days.

ACE inhibitors have complex effect and decrease blood pressure and plasma renin activity. The dramatic response to therapeutic inhibition of the renin-angiotensin system in SRC implicates renin overproduction as a central part of the pathogenesis of SRC [1, 42].

Several cohort studies showed benefit in survival with the use of ACE inhibitors in patients with SRC. The experts recommend immediate use of ACE inhibitors in the treatment of SRC [11, 17–19, 29, 43–48]. Prospective analysis of 108 patients with SRC has suggested that patients on ACE inhibitors (captopril in 47 and enalapril in 8) had a significantly better 1 year survival rate (76%) and 5 years (66%) compared to patients without ACE inhibitors (15% at one and 10% at 5 years, respectively). Treatment with ACE inhibitors was significantly associated with better survival in SRC, after adjustment for age and blood pressure ($p < 0.001$) [29, 49, 50]. Two recent retrospective studies including 91 and 110 patients with SRC, respectively, the majority of whom (91 and 98% respectively) were treated with ACE inhibitors and/or angiotensin receptor antagonists (ARA), reported survival rates from 71–82% at 1 year, 59–60% at 5 years, and 42–47% at 10 years [19, 47]. Other anti-hypertensive agents may be considered for management of refractory hypertension in conjunction with an ACE inhibitor in SRC, including ARA, calcium channel blockers, doxazosin, and clonidine [1, 49]. Beta-blockers are not appropriate, as they affect peripheral circulation.

It can be summarized that survival benefit was shown with the use of ACE inhibitors in patients with SRC. Experts recommend immediate use of ACE inhibitors in the treatment of SRC [17].

2.10.3.2 Acute kidney injury

A patient with SRC is, from a definition, the one with acute kidney injury and should be managed in cooperation with a nephrologist. Thus, recommendation for acute kidney injury should be applied including regular monitoring of kidney function, minimization of nephrotoxic medication, etc. During first days of SRC treatment, serum creatinine levels usually increase. This is an anticipated decrease in glomerular filtration that should not discourage us from intensive blood pressure control [27].

Renal replacement therapy should be initiated if necessary. Both hemodialysis and peritoneal dialysis are possible alternatives. However, hemodialysis is a preferred option. ACE inhibitor treatment should continue long term, even in patients on chronic renal replacement therapy, especially in patients with possible recovery of renal function.

In chronic hemodialysis patients, kidney transplantation has to be considered. There are two particular details in SSc patients that should be discussed: first, there is a possibility of late recovery of kidney function and, second, there is historically reported bad outcome of transplanted SSc patients. Indeed, patients with SRC may recover renal function up to 3 years after the crisis, most often within 12–18 months [50]. Thus, many authors recommend that decision to transplant should not be made before 2 years after SRC onset [17]. Patients after SRC on hemodialysis treatment should therefore be regularly checked for signs of recovery of kidney function. But in general, postponing kidney transplant in hemodialysis patients could worsen their prognosis. It seems prudent that in patients without significant residual renal function, without signs of kidney recovery and unfavorable findings on kidney biopsy (if done) such as vascular thrombosis and glomerular ischemic collapse, we consider kidney transplant in 6 months from SRC [51].

Older studies reported bad outcome of SSc patients after kidney transplant compared to patients with other causes of kidney failure. However, recent studies have shown excellent patient and graft survival [52].

Generally, on the other hand, long-term dialysis increases the risk of death. Independent of the underlying disease, dialysis increases the risk of infection (in patients undergoing peritoneal dialysis) and, over the long term, enhances the risk of vascular calcification and atherosclerosis. In patients on chronic dialysis, kidney transplantation has to be considered [53].

In a series of 260 SSc patients who underwent renal transplantation in the United States, their 5-year graft-survival rate was 56.7% [53]. In that study, the risk of SRC recurrence was higher for patients with early renal insufficiency following SRC onset. Recurrent SRC in the allograft may be predicted by the same previously described risk factors [53–55].

For those with recurrent SRC, the time of onset following transplantation is not known. Recurrence usually happens within the first few months to the first 1–2 years after transplantation [53, 54].

Kidney transplantation should therefore be considered in all SSc patients with the need of renal replacement therapy. What has not changed over the last decade is that only small percentage of patients with SSc is transplanted due to severe extrarenal disease. Thorough work-up before enrolling a patient on waiting list is warranted.

Both recurrence of SRC after kidney transplantation and graft loss due to SRC recurrence have been reported. Recurrence rate is fortunately low (8.8%) and patients after kidney transplant should be monitored similarly to patients with SSc at high risk of SRC development [52].

Immunosuppression given to SSc patients after kidney transplant alters the course of the disease. Most of the patients after kidney transplant have stable disease or even improve symptoms. Regarding immunosuppressive regimens after kidney transplant, it is difficult to make any evidence-based conclusions. Most patients were treated with high-dose steroids at the time of transplantation followed by long-term low doses in combination with calcineurin inhibitors and mycophenolate mofetil. A significant number of patients were weaned from steroids with reasonable outcome, but recommendations cannot be made due to limited number of patients [52].

2.10.3.3 Plasma exchange

Plasma exchange, which has been proposed for thrombotic microangiopathy, has not demonstrated efficacy and should not be prescribed, with the exception of the rare SRC patients who might develop thrombotic microangiopathy associated with anti-ADAMTS-13 antibodies [54]. There are no clinical trial data for use of plasma exchange in SRC.

3. Nonscleroderma renal crisis involvement of kidney in systemic sclerosis

3.1 Intersticial kidney changes/disease

Clinically relevant renal involvement (non-SRC) in SSc is uncommon [55]. Asymptomatic and slowly progressive renal involvement is present in 60–80% of SSc patients. In more than half of asymptomatic SSc patients, renal function demonstrates clinical markers of renal damage (proteinuria, elevation of serum creatinine, hypertension, etc.) [32, 56–58]. These patients presented with evidence of underlying chronic renal disease but without confounding illnesses such as diabetes or hypertension existing prior to the onset of their SSc. Histological findings showed expressions of fibrillar collagens. In some SSc cases, drug exposure may explain interstitial kidney changes [6]. It is unclear whether SSc cases are more susceptible to this, but interstitial nephritis remains an important differential diagnosis.

3.2 Glomerulonephritis

Glomerulonephritis occurs in the context of overlap connective tissue disease or systemic vasculitis. In other words, SSc should be associated with other immunopathological diseases presented by glomerulonephritis, mainly systemic lupus erythematosus and ANCA-associated glomerulonephritis [59].

Circulating antimyeloperoxidase antibodies have been reported in several patients with dcSSc associated with necrotizing and crescentic glomerulonephritis [1, 58]. A study of 81 SSc patients with renal impairment found 2 patients with lcSSc with perinuclear anti-neutrophil cytoplasmic antibodies (p-ANCA) along with circulating IgG and IgM antimyeloperoxidase antibodies. After screening for ANCA in SSc by indirect immunofluorescence, the levels of IgM and IgG anti-MPO antibodies in 8 patients (8%) with SSc were determined by ELISA [60]. In conclusion, the presence of ANCA in SSc patients should predict ANCA-associated vasculitis. The treatment of these associated glomerulonephritis is managed according to the principles of treatment of the overlapping renal diseases (**Figure 8**).

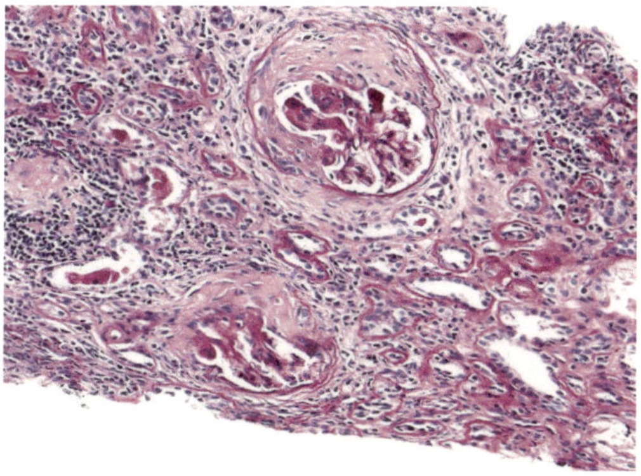

Figure 8.
Normotensive patient with systemic sclerosis and acute renal failure underwent renal biopsy. End-stage kidney disease: crescentic glomerulonephritis showing fibrous crescents. A mixed mononuclear cell infiltrate and considerable tubular loss are shown. Hematoxylin-eosin staining, magnification 200 times. Courtesy of Miroslav Podhola, MD., PhD., Department of Pathology, Faculty of Medicine in Hradec Kralove, Charles University.

4. Conclusion

SRC is a rare manifestation with dramatic clinical picture and high morbidity and mortality. Current strategies to reduce the associated morbidity and mortality include identification of at-risk patients to aid early diagnosis. Caution should be exercised in diagnosis of SSc cases with serological features of renal disease including anti-RNA polymerase III autoantibodies, for non-SRC renal disease SLE serology and ANCA positivity. ACE inhibitor therapy should be lifelong in all SRC patients. Prompt initiation of ACE inhibitors stays a key point in SRC therapy. New therapeutic possibilities are needed.

Acknowledgements

This work was supported by MH CZ—DRO UHHK, grant number 00179906; Charles University research projects [PROGRES Q40-15]; and MHCR 023728 and AZV-16-33542A.

Author details

Tomas Soukup[1*], Jan Toms[1], Sabina Oreska[2], Eva Honsova[3] and Roman Safranek[4]

1 Division of Rheumatology, 2nd Department of Gastroenterology, Charles University, Hradec Kralove, Czech Republic

2 Department of Rheumatology, Institute of Rheumatology, Charles University, Prague, Czech Republic

3 Department of Clinical and Transplant Pathology, Institute for Clinical and Experimental Medicine, Prague, Czech Republic

4 Division of Nephrology, Haemodialysis Centre, Charles University, Hradec Kralove, Czech Republic

*Address all correspondence to: tomas.soukup@fnhk.cz

References

[1] Denton CP, Hudson M. Renal crisis and other renal manifestation. In: Varga J, editor. Scleroderma. 2th ed. Londin, UK: Springer; 2017. pp. 317-330

[2] Nihtyanova SI, Schreiber BE, Ong VH, Rosenberg D, Moinzadeh P, Coghlan JG, et al. Prediction of pulmonary complications and long-term survival in systemic sclerosis. Arthritis & Rhematology. 2014;**66**(7):1625-1635

[3] Mouthon L, Bérezné A, Bussone G, Noël LH, Villiger PM, Guillevin L. Scleroderma renal crisis: A rare but severe complication of systemic sclerosis. Clinical Reviews in Allergy and Immunology. 2011;**40**(2):84-91

[4] Steen VD, Medsger TA. Changes in causes of death in systemic sclerosis, 1972-2002. Annals of the Rheumatic Diseases. 2007;**66**(7):940-944

[5] Tyndall AJ, Bannert B, Vonk M, et al. Causes and risk factors for death in systemic sclerosis: A study from the EULAR SclerodermaTrials and research (EUSTAR) database. Annals of the Rheumatic Diseases. 2010;**69**(10):1809-1815

[6] Bose N, Chiesa-Vottero A, Chatterjee S. Scleroderma renal crisis. Seminars in Arthritis and Rheumatism. 2015;**44**(6):687-694

[7] Batal I, Domsic RT, Medsger TA, Bastacky S. Scleroderma renal crisis: A pathology perspective. International Journal of Rheumatology. 2010;**20**(10):543-544

[8] Steen VD, Mayes MD, Merkel PA. Assessment of kidney involvement. Clinical and Experimental Rheumatology. 2003;**21**:S29-S31

[9] Butler EA, Baron M, Fogo AB, Frech T, Ghossein C, Hachulla E. Generation of a Core set of items to develop classification criteria for scleroderma renal CrisisUsing consensus methodology. Arthritis & Rhematology. 2019;**71**(6):964-971. DOI: 10.1002/art.40809. [Epub ahead of print]

[10] Hoa S, Stern EP, Denton CP, Hudson M. Scleroderma clinical trials consorcium scleroderma renal crisis working group investigators of the scleroderma clinical trials consortium scleroderma renal crisis working group. Towards developing criteria for scleroderma renal crisis: A scoping review. Autoimmunity Reviews. 2017;**16**(4):407-415

[11] Helfrich DJ, Banner B, Steen VD, et al. Normotensive renal failure in systemic sclerosis. Arthritis and Rheumatism. 1989;**32**(9):1128-1134

[12] Steen VD, Medsger TA Jr, Osial TA Jr, Ziegler GL, Shapiro AP, Rodnan GP. Factors predicting development of renal involvement in progressive systemic sclerosis. The American Journal of Medicine 1984;**76**(5):779-786

[13] Phan TG, Cass A, Gillin A, Trew P, Fertig N, Sturgess A. Anti-RNA polymerase III antibodies in the diagnosis of scleroderma renal crisis sine scleroderma. The Journal of Rheumatology. 1999;**26**(11):2489-2492

[14] Avouac J, Walker UA, Hachulla E, Riemekasten G, Cuomo G, Carreira PE, et al. Joint and tendon involvement predict disease progression in systemic sclerosis: A EUSTAR prospective study. Annals of the Rheumatic Diseases. 2016;**75**(1):103-109

[15] Steen VD, Medsger TA Jr. Case-control study of corticosteroids and other drugs that either precipitate or protect from the development of scleroderma renal crisis.Arthritis and Rheumatism 1998;**41**(9):1613-1619.

[16] Allanore Y, Meune C, Vonk MC, et al. Prevalence and factors associated with left ventricular dysfunction in the EULAR scleroderma trial and research group (EUSTAR) database patients with systemic sclerosis. Annals of the Rheumatic Diseases. 2010;**69**:218-221

[17] Kowal-Bielecka O, Fransen J, Avouac J, Becker M, Kulak A, Allanore Y, et al. Update of EULAR recommendations for the treatment of systemic sclerosis. Annals of the Rheumatic Diseases. 2017;**76**(8):1327-1339

[18] Teixeira L, Mouthon L, Mahr A, Berezné A, Agard C, Mehrenberger M, et al. Mortality and risk factors of scleroderma renal crisis: A French retrospective study of 50 patients. Annals of the Rheumatic Diseases. 2008;**67**(1):110-116

[19] Guillevin L, Bérezné A, Seror R, et al. Scleroderma renal crisis: A retrospective multicentre study on 91 patients and 427 controls. Rheumatology (Oxford). 2012;**51**(3):460-467

[20] DeMarco PJ, Weisman MH, Seibold JR, et al. Predictors and outcomes of scleroderma renal crisis: The high-dose versus low-dose D-penicillamine in early diffuse systemic sclerosis trial. Arthritis and Rheumatism. 2002;**46**(11):2983-2989

[21] Montanelli G, Beretta L, Santaniello A, et al. Effect of dihydropyridine calcium channel blockers and glucocorticoids on the prevention and development of scleroderma renal crisis in an Italian case series. Clinical and Experimental Rheumatology. 2013;**31**(Suppl 76):135-139

[22] Hesselstrand R, Scheja A, Wuttge DM. Scleroderma renal crisis in a Swedish systemic sclerosis cohort: Survival, renal outcome, and RNA polymerase III antibodies as a risk factor. Scandinavian Journal of Rheumatology. 2012;**41**(1):39-43

[23] Iudici M, Fasano S, Iacono D, Russo B, Cuomo G, Valentini G. Prevalence and factors associated with glucocorticoids (GC) use in systemic sclerosis (SSc): A systematic review and meta-analysis of cohort studies and registries. Clinical Rheumatology. 2014;**33**(2):153-164

[24] Takahashi T, Asano Y, Noda S, Aozasa N, Akamata K, Taniguchi T. A possible contribution of lipocalin-2 to the development of dermal fibrosis, pulmonary vascular involvement and renal dysfunction in systemic sclerosis. The British Journal of Dermatology. 2015;**173**(3):681-689

[25] Yanaba K, Asano Y, Tada Y, Sugaya M, Kadono T, Hamaguchi Y, et al. Increased serum soluble CD147 levels in patients with systemic sclerosis: Association with scleroderma renal crisis. Clinical Rheumatology. 2012;**31**(5):835-839

[26] Andreussi R, Silva LMB, da Silva HC, Luppino-Assad AP, Andrade DCO, Sampaio-Barros PD. Systemic sclerosis induced by the use of cocaine: Is there an association? Rheumatology International. 2019;**39**(2):387-393

[27] Kellum J, Lameire N, Aspelin P, Barsoum RS, Burdmann E, Goldstein SL, et al. KDIGO clinical practice guideline for acute kidney injury. Kidney International. Supplement. 2012;**2**(2):1-138

[28] Del Mercado VM, Topete MA, Aguilera BCR, De La Torre GI. Diffuse alveolar hemorrhage in limited cutaneous systemic sclerosis with positive perinuclear antineutrophil cytoplasmic antibodies. The Journal of Rheumatology. 1996;**23**(10):1821-1823

[29] Steen VD, Medsger TA Jr. Epidemiology and natural history

of systemic sclerosis. Rheumatic Diseases Clinics of North America. 1990;**16**(1):1-10

[30] Bunn CC, Denton CP, Shi-Wen X, Knight C, Black CM. Anti-RNA polymerases and other autoantibody specificities in systemic sclerosis. British Journal of Rheumatology. 1998;**37**(1):15-20

[31] Okano Y, Steen VD, Medsger TA Jr. Autoantibody reactive with RNA polymerase III in systemic sclerosis. Annals of Internal Medicine 1993;**119**(10):1005-1013

[32] Rivolta R, Mascagni B, Berruti V, Quarto DiPalo F, Elli A, Scorza R, et al. Renal vascular damage in systemic sclerosis patients without clinical evidence of nephropathy. Arthritis and Rheumatism. 1996;**39**(6):1030-1034

[33] Nguyen B, Assassi S, Arnett FC, Mayes MD. Association of RNA polymerase III antibodies with scleroderma renal crisis. The Journal of Rheumatology. 2010;**37**(5):1068

[34] Codullo V, Cavazzana I, Bonino C, Alpini C, Cavagna L, Cozzi F, et al. Serologic profile and mortality rates of scleroderma renal crisis in Italy. The Journal of Rheumatology. 2009;**36**(7):1464-1469

[35] Kuwana M, Medsger A. The clinical aspects of antibodies. In: Varga J, editor. Scleroderma. 2th ed. London, UK: Springer; 2017. pp. 207-220

[36] Kfoury Baz EM, Mahfouz RA, Masri AF, Jamaleddine GW. Thrombotic thrombocytopenic purpura in a case of scleroderma renal crisis treated with twice-daily therapeutic plasma exchange. Renal Failure. 2001;**23**(5):737-742

[37] Cervera R, Rodríguez-Pintó I, Colafrancesco S, Conti F, Valesini G, Rosário C, et al. 14th international congress on antiphospholipid antibodies task force report on catastrophic antiphospholipid syndrome. Autoimmunity Reviews. 2014;**13**(7):699-707

[38] Arnaud L, Huart A, Plaisier E, Francois H, Mougenot B, Tiev K, et al. ANCA-related crescentic glomerulonephritis in systemic sclerosis: Revisiting the "normotensive scleroderma renal crisis". Clinical Nephrology. 2007;**68**(3):165-170

[39] Silver MR, Denton CP. Case Studies in Systemic Sclerosis. London: Springer-Verlag London Limited; 2011. Print ISBN: 978-0-85729-640-5

[40] Hudson M, Baron M, Tatibouet S, Furst DE, Khanna D, Hummers L, et al. Exposure to ACE inhibitors prior to the onset of scleroderma renal crisis-results from the international scleroderma renal crisis survey. Seminars in Arthritis and Rheumatism. 2014;**43**(5):666-672

[41] Zanatta E, Polito P, Favaro M, Larosa M, Marson P, Cozzi F, et al. Therapy of scleroderma renal crisis: State of the art. Autoimmunity Reviews. 2018;**17**(9):882-889

[42] Sterm EP, Steen VD, Denton CP. Management of renal involvement in Scleroderma. Current Treatment Options in Rheumatology. 2015;**1**(1):06-81

[43] Woodworth TG, Suliman YA, Li W, Furst DE, Clements P. Scleroderma renal crisis and renal involvement in systemic sclerosis. Nature Reviews Nephrology. 2016;**12**(11):678-691

[44] Rossi D, Zanatta E, Marson P, Sciascia S, Polito P, Roccatello D, et al. How I treat patients with systemic sclerosis in clinical practice. Autoimmunity Reviews. 2017 Oct;**16**(10):1024-1028

[45] Lopez-Ovejero JA, Saal SD, D'Angelo WA, et al. Reversal of vascular and renal crises of scleroderma by oral angiotensin-converting-enzyme blockade. The New England Journal of Medicine. 1979;**300**(25):1417-1419

[46] Steen VD, Medsger TA Jr. Long-term outcomes of scleroderma renal crisis. Annals of Internal Medicine 2000;**133**(8):600-603

[47] Penn H, Howie AJ, Kingdon EJ, Bunn CC, Stratton RJ, Black CM, et al. Scleroderma renal crisis: Patient characteristics and long-term outcomes. QJM. 2007;**100**(8):485-494

[48] Kowal-Bielecka O, Landewé R, Avouac J, Chwiesko S, Miniati I, Czirjak L, et al. EULAR recommendations for the treatment of systemic sclerosis: A report from the EULAR scleroderma trials and research group (EUSTAR). Annals of the Rheumatic Diseases. 2009;**68**(5):620-628

[49] Nagaraja V, Denton CP, Khanna D. Old medications and new targeted therapies in systemic sclerosis. Rheumatology (Oxford). 2015;**54**(11):1944-1953

[50] Lynch BM, Stern EP, Ong V, Harber M, Burns A, Denton CP. UK scleroderma study group (UKSSG) guidelines on the diagnosis and management of scleroderma renal crisis. Clinical and Experimental Rheumatology. 2016;**34 Suppl 100**(5):106-109

[51] Shanmugam VK, Steen VD. Renal disease in scleroderma: An update on evaluation, risk stratification, pathogenesis and management. Current Opinion in Rheumatology. 2012;**24**(6):669-676

[52] Bertrand D et al. Kidney transplantation in patients with systemic sclerosis: A nationwide multicentre study. Transplant International. 2017;**30**:256-265

[53] Guillevin L, Mouthon L. Scleroderma Renal Crisis. Rheumatic Diseases Clinics of North America. 2015;**41**(3):475-488

[54] Pham PT, Pham PC, Danovitch GM, et al. Predictors and risk factors for recurrent scleroderma renal crisis in the kidney allograft: Case report and review of the literature. American Journal of Transplantation. 2005;**5**(10):2565-2569

[55] Galluccio F, Müller-Ladner U, Furst DE, Khanna D, Matucci-Cerinic M. Points to consider in renal involvement in systemic sclerosis. Rheumatology (Oxford). 2017;**56**(suppl_5):v49-v52

[56] Bussone G, Bérezné A, Pestre V, Guillevin L, Mouthon L. The scleroderma kidney: Progress in risk factors, therapy, and prevention. Current Rheumatology Reports. 2011;**13**(1):37-43

[57] Shanmugam VK, Steen VD. Renal manifestations in scleroderma: Evidence for subclinical renal disease as a marker of vasculopathy. International Journal of Rheumatology. 2010;**20**(10):538-539

[58] Livi R, Guiducci S, Perfetto F, et al. Lack of activation of renal functional reserve predicts the risk of significant renal involvement in systemic sclerosis. Annals of the Rheumatic Diseases. 2011;**70**(8):196-197

[59] Kamen DL, Wigley FM, Brown AN. Antineutrophil cytoplasmic antibodypositive crescentic glomerulonephritis in scleroderma-a different kind of renal crisis. The Journal of Rheumatology. 2006;**33**(5):1886-1888

[60] Locke IC, Worrall JG, Leaker B, Black CM, Cambridge G. Autoantibodies to myeloperoxidase in systemic sclerosis. The Journal of Rheumatology. 1997;**24**(5):86-89

Chapter 3

Gastrointestinal Involvement in Systemic Sclerosis: Overview, Neglected Aspects, Malnutrition, Body Composition and Management

Sabina Oreska and Michal Tomcik

Abstract

Gastrointestinal tract (GIT) involvement is the most common internal organ manifestation and is present in up to 90% of patients with systemic sclerosis (SSc). Clinical manifestations can differ according to the part of the GIT affected, disease course and symptoms. A majority of the symptoms are caused by GIT dysmotility. Up to 8% of SSc patients develop several GIT symptoms, which increase the mortality. Although GIT involvement is rarely the direct cause of death, it can lead to several comorbidities including malnutrition and negative alterations of body composition. These factors have a negative impact on quality of life and increase the mortality. To date, the treatment is rather symptomatic. The pathogenesis of GIT involvement in SSc still remains to be clarified to improve the treatment approaches including intravenous immunoglobulins and microRNA interventions.

Keywords: gastrointestinal tract, systemic sclerosis, malnutrition, body composition, diagnosis, management

1. Introduction

Systemic sclerosis (SSc), characterised by autoimmune inflammation, vasculopathy and fibrotic tissue deposition as the main pathophysiological features, can affect any organ system. In fact, the aetiology and pathophysiology of SSc are still not completely elucidated [1]. Gastrointestinal tract (GIT) is one of the most commonly involved organ systems in SSc.

Up to 90% of SSc patients are affected by some degree of GIT fibrosis, with no difference in frequency in limited cutaneous systemic sclerosis (lcSSc) and diffuse cutaneous systemic sclerosis (dcSSc) subsets. However, more severe involvement and increased mortality occur rather in dcSSc than lcSSc [2, 3]. Dysmotility is the cardinal pathological abnormality, which can affect any part of GIT and contributes to the majority of symptoms [4], which are mostly non-specific and overlapping for a particular anatomical site. GIT involvement varies in extent, severity and course and can manifest even in the absence of cutaneous disease [5].

The pathophysiology of GIT involvement in general corresponds to the skin and other organ involvement in SSc, with the main characteristic pathologic features: vascular abnormalities, immune cell infiltration in tissue, autoantibodies and typical extensive deposition of collagen fibres. This process leads to specific early myenteric neural dysfunction caused by autoantibodies and collagen deposition, vasculopathy in myointimal layer mainly in capillaries preceding the muscle changes, smooth muscle cell infiltration with mononuclear cells with consequent atrophy and fibrosis of enteric connective tissue [1, 6]. Regarding the aetiology, genetic component is supposed to play a significant role in GIT involvement. In the Canadian population study, in which SSc patents were classified according to the ethnicity, population of white patients had less severe GIT involvement compared to North American native population (including American Indians and others), suggesting a predisposition for severity and progression of the disease [7]. Another study identified some haplotypes in an American native population (Choctaw Indians) strongly associated with SSc and more severe progression of this disease (HLA-DRB1*1602, DQB1*0301 and DQA1*0501) [8]. Some studies have also reported high prevalence of *Helicobacter* infection in SSc patients, supporting the hypothesis of infectious aetiology [9]. Smoking has been identified as the only environmental factor associated with increased severity of GIT symptoms in SSc [10].

GIT involvement significantly impacts quality of life and contributes to depression, sleep disturbance and pain [11–13]. It also negatively influences the prognosis with up to 12% of mortality due to fibrosis of GIT and accompanying malnutrition [1]. Up to 8% of SSc patients can develop severe GIT symptoms, which lead to increased mortality with only 15% survival at 9 years [5].

2. Pathophysiology

The pathophysiology of GIT involvement in SSc is a complex process. Unfortunately, it is still poorly understood due to many reasons: heterogeneity of clinical manifestations, the lack of appropriate animal models and the paucity of studies examining the pathophysiology. The key pathogenic mechanisms of GIT involvement, similarly to SSc in general, include fibro-proliferative vasculopathy, immune dysfunction with the participation of various components of immune system and fibrosis [14].

Endothelial injury as the crucial event in SSc results in increased production of reactive oxygen species (ROS) and release of chemokines and growth factors. Recruited immune cells (B- and T-cells and pro-fibrotic macrophages) contribute to further release of ROS, cytokines and pro-fibrotic mediators [15]. These mechanisms lead to reduced blood flow in mucosa, endothelial cell apoptosis, perivascular infiltrates and thickening of the basement membrane [16–18].

The initial step in pathophysiology of GIT dysmotility is neuropathy, followed by myopathy and later by progress to fibrosis [19]. Specific autoantibodies isolated from serum of SSc patients (SSc-IgGs) were described to cause significant smooth muscle dysfunction [20]. The mechanism lies in inhibition of acetylcholine binding on the M3 receptors (M3-Rs) [21, 22]. The action of SSc-IgGs seems to be dependent on the disease stage: in early SSc there is higher affinity of SSc-IgGs to the M3-Rs of myenteric neurons, which represents the neuropathic damage. During the course of the disease, the affinity increases to both smooth muscle cells and myenteric neurons, representing the myopathic phase. This temporal increase of SSc-IgGs affinity could elucidate the progressive character of GIT involvement [14, 19, 23].

Presence and action of M3-R autoantibodies can explain the impaired GIT function explored by manometry before the occurrence of histological changes [14].

Neutralisation of M3-R antibodies by human intravenous immunoglobulins (IVIGs) and its antigen-binding fragment F(ab)2 might reverse the intestinal dysfunction and is considered as a potential therapy [19]. The ultimate smooth muscle cell atrophy and tissue fibrosis lead to the loss of GIT contractile function and disability to respond to any external stimuli; thus any treatment of dysmotility is futile [14].

Alterations in cell-mediated immunity have a significant role in SSc GIT involvement [24, 25]. Interleukin (IL)-4 stimulates type 2 helper (Th2) polarisation of CD4+ T-cells, which is predominant in SSc. Th2 cells further upregulate humoral immunity [15, 26]. CD4+ T-cells in immune cell infiltrates in gastric biopsy specimens with typically increased CD4+/CD8+ T-cell ratio can be responsible for pathogenic autoantibody production and fibrosis of GIT [14, 27]. Generalised fibrosis with increased deposition of collagens I and III in most layers (muscularis mucosae, submucosa and muscularis propria) was described in gastric wall biopsies, together with strong expression of fibrogenic cytokines (transforming growth factor-β and connective tissue growth factor) and α-smooth muscle actin [28]. Other factors contributing to fibrosis are reduction of matrix metalloproteinase-1 expression and damage and reduction of telocytes—specific stromal cells essential for extracellular matrix scaffolding [29, 30]. Moreover, consequent increased stiffness of GIT wall is an additional potential stimulus for further fibrosis [31].

In addition, differentially expressed microRNAs (miRNAs) targeting both inflammation and fibrotic pathways have a probable role in SSc pathogenesis [32, 33]. Depletion of the miR-29 family, which targets collagen gene expression and regulates fibrosis, probably leads to increased collagen deposition in tissues [34].

3. Clinical manifestations

As mentioned, any part of GIT can be affected, so the clinical manifestations vary according to the involved organ. Large proportion of patients are asymptomatic, or symptoms may be unspecific and overlapping [1]. Fibrosis and dysfunction of GIT lead to many complications, such as gastro-oesophageal reflux disease (GERD) with complications (oesophageal strictures, Barrett's oesophagus), dilation and non-compliance of the stomach (gastroparesis), small intestinal bacterial overgrowth (SIBO), colonic dilation and dysfunction of internal anal sphincter. The vasculopathic manifestations are gastric antral vascular ectasia (GAVE), small intestine vascular ectasia and diverticula in the oesophagus, small intestine and colon, resulting in malabsorption and faecal incontinence [14]. Clinical features are divided according to individual organ involvement.

3.1 Oral cavity and pharynx

There are numerous SSc-related alterations of the oral cavity [35]. Pathognomic fibrosis results in characteristically reduced oral aperture (microstomia), thickening of the sublingual fraenulum and widening of periodontal ligaments [36]. In addition, secondary Sjögren's syndrome, reported in about one fifth of SSc patients, can lead to tooth loss along with above-mentioned pathologies. All these factors complicate dental hygiene and food intake and contribute to malnutrition [37]. Up to 20% of SSc patients can develop mandibular resorption predisposing to pathological fractures, osteomyelitis and trigeminal neuralgia [38]. Oropharyngeal dysphagia manifests in 25% of SSc patients and is caused both by dysmotility and GER as a reflex mechanism [39]. Apart from malnutrition, dysphagia is also a risk factor for aspiration pneumonia [40]. With regard to malignancy, risk of tongue cancer (squamous cell carcinoma) has been reported in dcSSc 25-fold higher compared to general population [41].

3.2 Oesophagus

Oesophageal dysfunction appears to be the most common GIT manifestation in SSc affecting up to 90% SSc patients with higher prevalence and tendency to deteriorate over time in dcSSc compared to lcSSc [42, 43]. Up to 30% of SSc patients may suffer from asymptomatic oesophageal involvement [44]. The main feature of oesophageal involvement is dysphagia due to smooth muscle cell atrophy and destruction of neuronal complexes. Drug-induced dysphagia and *Candida* oesophagitis caused by immunosuppressive treatment should be also taken into account. Reduced lower oesophageal sphincter (LES) tone along with dilation of the lumen, peristalsis disorder and gastroparesis is the main predisposing factor for GERD and consequent complications. Among typical symptoms asthma should not be omitted when taking patient's history [14, 42].

Long-standing GERD results in development of distal reflux oesophagitis and eventually progresses to peptic strictures and Barrett's oesophagus (BE) formation. The prevalence of BE is reported to be 12.7% in SSc patients treated with proton-pump inhibitors (PPIs) [45]. Approximately 20% of these patients develop dysplasia and are at higher risk of adenocarcinoma compared to SSc patients with BE and without dysplasia. However, this risk seems not to be increased in SSc compared to general population with GERD [45, 46].

The recent high-resolution manometry study reported positive correlation of severe oesophageal dysmotility with the duration of SSc and presence of interstitial lung disease (ILD) [47]. GERD can contribute to the emergence of ILD and worsen the ILD in SSc by microaspiration of gastric content; therefore, early diagnosis and administration of high-dose PPI therapy are needed [48, 49].

3.3 Stomach

Gastric involvement leads mainly to gastroparesis and GAVE [50]. Gastroparesis manifests clinically by early satiety, nausea and vomiting, epigastric discomfort and bloating and may progress to complete food intolerance [51, 52]. GAVE, also called "watermelon stomach", is considered a macroscopic manifestation of SSc vasculopathy, corresponds with skin telangiectasias and is associated with Raynaud's phenomenon [53, 54]. The prevalence of GAVE in SSc ranges from 6 to 22% [53–56]. It usually occurs within the first few years from the onset of the disease. Nevertheless, it can also be the first SSc manifestation in the absence of cutaneous involvement, clinically expressed as anaemia of combined aetiology: iron deficiency (sideropenia) and chronic bleeding (occult bleeding, melena or haematemesis) [56]. The presence of GAVE correlated negatively with the positivity of anti-topoisomerase I antibodies, but, in one study, was not associated with anti-RNA polymerase III autoantibodies (anti-RNAP3) [54]. However, on contrary, an association was confirmed in the recent study of EUSTAR population, where 48% of patients with GAVE had anti-RNAP3 positivity compared to 16% of SSc patients without GAVE. Of note, the autoantibody profile was not available for the whole cohort of SSc patients included [57]. A more recent study of EUSTAR population including almost 5000 SSc patients assessing the association of anti-RNAP3 autoantibodies with clinical features and risk of malignancies reported, among other results, a negative association of anti-RNAP3 with GERD and a positive association of anti-RNAP3 with GAVE (more than eight times increased risk of GAVE in anti-RNAP3-positive patients than in anti-RNAP3-negative SSc patients) [58]. The association with specific antibodies and its potential clinical use is a quest for further studies.

3.4 Small intestine

The small intestine belongs to the most commonly affected organ of GIT involvement in SSc, after the oesophagus and anorectum. Decreased motility results in typical complications, which participate in malabsorption and malnutrition: local small bowel dilation, intestinal pseudo-obstruction and SIBO, development of pneumatosis cystoides intestinalis (PCI) and jejunal diverticula [59]. The range of symptoms is wide, from dyspeptic symptoms to systemic symptoms resulting from malabsorption [14].

Predisposing factors for pseudo-obstruction, either acute or chronic, are both SSc related—dilation, atony and delayed transit—and treatment related, especially the use of opiates [51, 60]. The stasis due to dysmotility of intestinal content predisposes to SIBO that was detected in up to 40–50% of SSc patients [51, 61]. This can, along with the failure of recurrent antibiotics therapy, cause the vulnerability to severe malabsorption [62].

PCI is a rare complication of SSc characterised by multiple gas-filled cysts in submucosa or subserosa [63] as an incidental radiographic (RDG) finding. Contributing factors involve dysmotility with consequent SIBO, ischemic damage and muscular atrophy [64]. Rarely, the rupture can cause benign spontaneous pneumoperitoneum or more severe complications as bowel ischaemia, perforation and peritonitis [63]. The treatment of benign pneumoperitoneum consists of conservative approach (oxygen, antibiotics and bowel rest) or surgery intervention in more severe cases [14].

3.5 Large intestine

Colonic involvement, including hypomotility, telangiectasia and diverticula, affects up to 50% of SSc patients and is often asymptomatic or can typically manifest by chronic constipation and abdominal distension [1]. Dysmotility and the resulting constipation can in extreme cases lead to faecal impaction or perforation requiring surgery. The colon can be dilated with the loss of haustration [14]. SSc patients can also suffer from diarrhoea and severe malabsorption caused by SIBO [65].

Colon and anorectal involvement can manifest by rectal prolapse and diverticula typically described as "wide mouth", which are mostly asymptomatic and not complicated by diverticulitis. Anorectal involvement is regarded as the second most common with a prevalence of 50–70% [14]. Symptoms include incontinence, tenesmus and painful defaecation. Faecal incontinence, present in 40% SSc patients, is generally attributable to several factors: diarrhoea, internal and external anal sphincter dysfunction, reduced rectal compliance and capacity with impaired recto-anal inhibitory reflex, rectal prolapse and also constipation with overflow [66, 67]. Dysfunction of smooth muscles in internal anal sphincter (neuropathic or myopathic) is supposed to be the initial cause of faecal incontinence [68]. The main cause of sphincter involvement seems to be the vasculopathy and resulting tissue atrophy described in endo-anal ultrasound imaging as a hyperechoic thinned sphincter. On the other hand, thick hypoechoic sphincter due to tissue fibrosis is found in some cases [69].

3.6 Liver and pancreas

Involvement of the liver is less frequent compared to GIT organs mentioned above. Nodular regenerative hyperplasia (NRH), benign liver involvement in SSc, can precede primary biliary cirrhosis (PBC) and can progress to non-cirrhotic portal hypertension [70, 71]. The pathogenesis lies in obliterative changes in portal veins and corresponds with the microvascular damage in SSc. Although NRH is mostly asymptomatic, it can develop into portal hypertension [72].

Primary biliary cirrhosis is the most common liver disorder associated with SSc with a prevalence of about 2%, higher in lcSSc [73]. It can precede the diagnosis of SSc, for example, as a Reynolds syndrome comprising PBC with Raynaud's phenomenon [74]. PBC is associated with anti-centromere antibody positivity [73]. Nevertheless, PBC screening antibodies (anti-mitochondrial, anti-gp21, anti-sp100) are detectable also in 20% of SSc patients with no liver disease [75]. The rate of progression of SSc-related PBC to end-stage liver disease and transplantation is lower compared to non-SSc PBC, but the reason is still unknown [76]. PBC contributes via cholestasis and decreased bile acid secretion to malabsorption and malnutrition [1].

Other rare liver infections in SSc include autoimmune hepatitis, idiopathic portal hypertension and primary sclerosing cholangitis [77, 78]. Specific anti-liver kidney microsomal (anti-LKM) or anti-smooth muscle (anti-SMA) antibodies detected in SSc without liver involvement are attributable to the autoimmune character of SSc [79].

The involvement of the pancreas seems to be rare and the symptoms can overlap with SIBO. The exocrine pancreatic insufficiency can take part in malabsorption [80]. Case reports describe occlusion of medium-sized pancreatic arteries in SSc resulting in haemorrhagic pancreatitis and fatal pancreatic infarction [81].

4. Malnutrition

Prevalence of malnutrition in SSc patients is estimated to be 15–58% [51, 82, 83]. Mortality is significantly increased in underfed SSc patients compared to patients with adequate nutritional intakes, whereas about 4% deaths are attributable to consequences of malnutrition [14, 83]. Both GIT involvement and cachexia from chronic inflammation play a key role in malnutrition [51]. However, there are other additional risk factors for malnutrition worth mentioning, e.g. depression and anxiety, although their significance is uncertain [1, 84].

According to the data from the Canadian Scleroderma Research Group database on almost 600 SSc patients, malnutrition correlates with disease duration and severity, severity of anaemia, abdominal distension and the rate of subjective complains [51]. The American Society of Parenteral and Enteral Nutrition (ASPEN) recommends early screening for malnutrition in every patient with newly diagnosed SSc and then annually [85]. Screening is performed by examination of blood samples for chosen parameters: haemoglobin, iron and vitamin B12, serum levels of fat-soluble vitamins, prealbumin, albumin and additional test for micro- and macronutrient deficiency, particularly in suspected SIBO [86].

Patients at risk are indicated to rigorous monitoring and prompt treatment optimally in cooperation with dietitian and gastroenterologist [85]. At the advanced stage, nasoenteral feeding should be tried, eventually a percutaneous endoscopic gastrostomy or jejunostomy in case of severe gastroparesis. The last-mentioned approach carries the advantage of reduction of pulmonary aspiration risk. The most severe refractory intestinal involvement is indicated to parenteral nutrition (PN) [14].

5. Alterations of body composition

Negative changes of bone mineral density (BMD), weight loss and muscle atrophy are associated with the nutrition insufficiency, but can also be related to reduced ability of physical activities, and severity of the disease. There are only few studies investigating alterations of body composition (BC) in SSc. Up to date, no large study or meta-analysis is available. Studies mostly used dual-energy X-ray absorptiometry, which is a suitable method for measuring BMD, lean body mass (LBM) and fat mass (FM) [87].

Studies have reported reduced BMD, which is determined by many factors: malnutrition and vitamin D deficiency, decreased physical activity, corticosteroid and immunosuppressive treatment and the disease-specific features [88, 89]. Low circulating levels of vitamin D may be related to the extent of skin involvement [90].

Studies on BC including body mass index (BMI) and other methods are scarce and their results differ. One study describes no alterations of FM or LBM in SSc patients compared to control population [90]. On the contrary, another study reported significantly lower BMI, LBM and FM as well as lower BMD in SSc women compared to healthy women, whereas more significant alterations of BC were expressed in dcSSc [91]. BMI significantly negatively correlated with duration of the disease in SSc patients, which was also the only risk factor associated with low LBM (sarcopenia). Of interest, reported negative changes of BC were not associated with current dietary customs [91].

One study reported decreased left ventricular mass (LVM) evaluated by echocardiography as a potential marker of malnutrition, whereas LVM correlated positively with BMI and severity of vascular involvement but negatively with skin thickening [92]. Another study reported the correlation of visceral abdominal fat with the main cardiovascular risk factors [93]. Both these studies are lacking a control group.

There is a strong need for large, well-designed studies including complex methods for evaluation of BC and disease-specific features and an adequate control group, so that the consequences of BC alterations could be properly elucidated and managed.

6. Diagnostic tools

Every patient diagnosed with SSc should be referred to a gastroenterologist, even if asymptomatic regarding GIT involvement [14]. Problematic swallowing and oral pathology should be examined by other specialists (dentists, speech pathologists and eventually an oral surgeon) [1]. Social and psychosocial factors have certain impacts on some GIT symptoms and hence should be taken into consideration too.

A wide spectrum of investigation methods is available for detection of GIT involvement, including laboratory and imaging methods [14]. Endoscopy has a key role in evaluation of oesophageal and gastric involvement and is used for therapeutic interventions as well. Except for video endoscopy, manometry and pH test are also useful in testing dysmotility and reflux (especially refractory GERD) [86, 94]. Barium oesophagogram is indicated for detection of suspect strictures [95]. Barrett's oesophagus requires regular screening by endoscopic biopsies with frequency depending on the baseline finding: no initial dysplasia should be screened every 3–5 years, and low-grade or high-grade dysplasia is recommended for control screening every 3–6 months. Endoscopy is also indicated in anaemia due to suspected GAVE [86]. Gastroparesis should be confirmed by RDG (delayed gastric emptying), before administration of prokinetics [96]. Endoscopy in small intestinal involvement (e.g. capsule endoscopy) is restricted and difficult, particularly if dysmotility is the main symptom.

Diagnosis of SIBO is based on subjective complains and objective signs of malabsorption—weight loss and nutrient deficiency—confirmed by results of blood test showing low serum carotene level (marker of vitamin A absorption), low vitamin B12, 25-hydroxyvitamin D, iron, pathologic prothrombin time, etc. [86]. Though breath test has good specificity, the sensitivity is poor (65–70%) and is not able to detect bacterial overgrowth in more distal parts of the small intestine [97, 98]. Invention of appropriate diagnostic tools for evaluation of SIBO is still an unmet need.

7. Patient-reported outcomes

Validation and measurement of the consequences and outcomes related to certain disease and involvement can be challenging. Construction of appropriate questionnaires for evaluating SSc patients' symptoms and correlating them to objective disease features was the task in the last decade [14]. The first questionnaire assessing the overall severity and quality of life in the context of GIT involvement was the Scleroderma Gastrointestinal Tract 1.0 (SSC-GIT 1.0), validated in 2009 [99]. Later it was revised, shortened and adapted into final version called University of California, Los Angeles Scleroderma Clinical Trial Consortium GIT 2.0 (UCLA SCTC GIT 2.0) [100]. This revised questionnaire consists of 33 items taken from SSC-GIT 1.0 and 1 new item evaluating rectal incontinence (faecal soilage). Total GIT score correlates with the overall burden of GIT disease in SSc patients [100].

Another instrument developed by the National Institutes of Health is called Patient-Reported Outcome Measurement Information System (PROMIS) GI symptom item [101]. Compared to UCLA SCTC GIT 2.0, PROMIS contains more items and has additional scales for disrupted swallowing, nausea and vomiting. There is large correlation and satisfactory reliability between this two instruments, but PROMIS seems to be more easily comprehensible for general and low-literacy population, usable across diverse populations and less demanding for respondents to fulfil [102]. The only validated tool for evaluating the malnutrition in SSc patients is Malnutrition Universal Screening Tool (MUST) [103]. MUST is one of screening tools recommended by North American expert panel for initial screening of malnutrition in SSc patients, as it is easy to administer [85]. MUST reflects the weight change and acute dietary intake and can be less sensitive to nutritional status and GIT involvement than another tool Subject's Global Assessment (SGA) [104]. Although MUST can identify the severity of malnutrition in SSs, it does not reflect the symptomatology contributing to this problem [105]. MUST is generally recommended as the screening tool for nutritional status by several groups (*European Society* for Clinical Nutrition and Metabolism, ESPEN; National Institute for Health and Care Excellence, NICE; and North American expert panel [106].

8. Therapy

8.1 Current therapeutic options

To date, no specific disease-modifying drugs exist to stop the progress of the disease. Early diagnosis of SSc organ involvement is essential for symptomatic organ-specific treatment, until the irreversible fibrotic and hardly treatable damage develops [14]. Currently, treatment of SSc-related gastrointestinal involvement is based on symptomatic therapy and includes acid-reducing therapy and administration of antibiotics and prokinetics. Octreotide is prescribed in refractory small intestinal pseudo-obstruction and bacterial overgrowth [40, 107] (**Table 1**).

Manifestation of GIT involvement	**Initial therapy/examination**	**Other therapeutic approaches and lifestyle modifications**
GERD	Modification of diet and lifestyle PPI (daily administration)	1) Take PPI at least 30 minutes prior to eating; control the right intake 2) Consider increasing the dose of PPI—twice a day—or change the PPI drug 3) Add an H2 blocker at night 4) If symptoms are still present, perform pH-metry or endoscopy Lifestyle and diet modification: Small meals more frequently during the day, more food in the first half of the day; take a walk after eating; restrict from aggravating foods; sleep with the upper half of the body elevated or lay on the left side
Barrett's oesophagus	Optimal therapy of GERD, monitoring by a gastroenterologist, regular upper endoscopy	Radiofrequency ablation (RFA)—consider in low- or moderate-grade dysplasia, always indicated in high-grade dysplasia
Stricture	Optimal therapy of GERD	Consider endoscopic dilation, in case of persistent dysplasia
Gastroparesis	Prokinetics (after gastric emptying study to confirm delayed gastric emptying)	1) Modification of diet (small meals, walking after meal), adequate liquid intake 2) Metoclopramide (ECG monitoring due to risk of prolonged QT interval) 3) Domperidone or erythromycin (if QT interval is normal) 4) Treatment of nausea
GAVE	Firstly, upper endoscopy to verify the diagnosis; argon plasma therapy in case of active bleeding; support therapy in case of bleeding (red blood cell transfusion, etc.)	1) Repeated sessions of argon plasma therapy 2) Laser therapy as an alternative approach 3) Immunosuppressive therapy in indicated cases
SIBO	Breath test (poor sensitivity) Examination of malabsorption (laboratory tests, body composition) Therapeutic trial with antibiotics (metronidazole, ciprofloxacin, neomycin, rifaximin, amoxicillin, doxycycline)	1) Administration of antibiotics for 2 weeks—in recurrent cases repeat cyclic antibiotics therapy 2) Probiotics 3) Enteral or parenteral nutritional support 4) FODMAP diet*
Intestinal pseudo-obstruction	Clinical assessment Imaging examination to exclude the mechanical cause of obstruction (X-ray, CT) Initial therapy and nutritional support during the hospitalisation	1) Nutritional support 2) Prokinetics (subcutaneous octreotide) 3) Broad-spectrum antibiotics 4) Surgery (in resistant cases, to provide decompression)
Malnutrition	Regular screening, BMI examination, recommended screening tools (MUST) Laboratory markers of malnutrition	1) Nutritional support 2) (Total) parenteral nutrition 3) Percutaneous feeding tubes (endoscopy gastrostomy)

Manifestation of GIT involvement	Initial therapy/examination	Other therapeutic approaches and lifestyle modifications
Constipation	"Bowel hygiene" (adequate liquid and fibre intake), defaecation in timely manner, taking regular exercise or other physical activity	Osmotic laxatives, stool softeners
Diarrhoea	Firstly, identify the cause of diarrhoea (other than SSc or multifactorial)	Management of the cause of diarrhoea (dysmotility, SIBO, fat malabsorption, etc.)
Faecal incontinence	Management of diarrhoea and SIBO, biofeedback, pelvic-floor exercises	Sacral nerve stimulation in resistant cases

**FODMAP foods: inappropriate and irritating ingredients in patients with irritable bowel syndrome or chronic bowel disease (idiopathic bowel inflammation, celiac disease, etc.); FODMAP diet consists of eliminating the intake of these foods: fermentable oligosaccharides (gluten, onion, garlic, etc.), disaccharides (lactose), monosaccharides (fructose) and polyols (alcohol sugars)—these are poorly absorbable carbohydrates in the small intestine.*
Adapted from Ref. [86]; Abbreviations: GIT, gastrointestinal tract; GERD, gastro-oesophageal reflux disease; PPIs, proton-pump inhibitors; ECG, electrocardiogram; GAVE, gastric antral vascular ectasia, SIBO, small intestinal bacterial overgrowth; CT, computed tomography; BMI, body mass index; MUST, Malnutrition Universal Screening Tool

Table 1.
Therapeutic intervention and follow-up of SSc patients with GIT involvement

Firstly, non-pharmacological treatment—lifestyle modification—should be applied to improve symptoms: elevation of the head or upper half of the body in the bed, sleeping on the left side, modification of eating regimen (indigestion of multiple small meals during the day, avoidance of eating meal less than 3 or 4 hours before bedtime), loss of weight if obesity, cessation of smoking and minimalizing alcohol intake, avoidance of drinking beverages and taking food or drugs decreasing the LES pressure (caffeine drinks, chocolate, calcium channel blockers, nitrates) and appropriate education about using risk drugs (bisphosphonates, tetracycline, iron, NSAIDs) [86].

The last update of EULAR recommendations published in 2017 has summarised the up-to-date treatment management into three points: (1) PPI for treatment of SSc-related GERD and prevention of oesophageal ulcers, strictures and other adverse consequences, (2) prokinetics for control of the GIT dysmotility and (3) intermittent or rotating cycles of antibiotics for treatment of symptomatic SIBO. However, large randomised control trial (RCT) studies evaluating the above-mentioned medication in SSc are lacking [108].

A small RCT reported favourable effect of PPI on improvement of upper GIT symptoms in SSc [109]. Moreover, omeprazole potentially reduces or regresses the oesophageal fibrosis [110, 111]. On the other hand, long-term therapy with PPI potentially decreases the intestinal absorption and thus causes nutritional deficiency. It is associated with the risk of bacterial overgrowth and infections (*C. difficile*) and more adverse effects (cardiovascular disease, malignancy, dementia, etc.) [112]. H2 receptor antagonists (H2RA) are prescribed as the next step in GERD treatment, either in monotherapy or in combination with PPI [113]. H2RA control mainly the nocturnal histamine-dependent acid secretion, which is refractory to PPI [86].

Treatment by prokinetics is based on individual symptoms of GIT dysmotility and potential benefit to risk [108]. Several non-randomised or uncontrolled studies reported improvement of GI symptoms in SSc [107, 114–116]. Prokinetics improve refractory GERD symptoms via supporting the gastric emptying in cases of gastroparesis in patients treated adequately for GERD. Combination with antiemetics is favourable [86]. Inclusion of prokinetics in combination therapy may have benefits in the early disease stage. Nevertheless, there is only a little or no profit from using prokinetics in later stages with dominant smooth muscle atrophy [96]. Choice of a certain drug from this group depends on individual benefit for each patient [86]. Small studies in patients with SSc and other connective tissue diseases reported a beneficial effect of cisapride [117–121]. However, cisapride can cause long QT syndrome predisposing to severe arrhythmias; thus it is not commonly available in some countries [122]. Metoclopramide is the first-line therapy in gastroparesis, followed by domperidone, erythromycin, or eventually pyridostigmine. Using these medicaments also requires monitoring for adverse effects [86].

In patients suspected for SIBO, intermittent or rotating administration of antibiotics is indicated. The current approach is based on empirical courses of one or more broad-spectrum antibiotics [123]. A therapeutic trial is performed for 2 weeks, without any testing. After these courses of antibiotics, gastrointestinal symptoms are assessed and if there is no improvement, cyclical courses of antibiotics continue every 2 weeks altered by 2 weeks off [86]. Therapy duration and regimen depend on the severity and recurrence of symptoms and clinical response [86]. Two small studies reported favourable effect of antibiotics in SSc-related SIBO [61, 124]. Nutritional status should not be omitted, and the supplementation should be eventually started at the same time as antibiotics [86]. Probiotics have favourable effect on symptoms and are suitable also in combination with antibiotics [125, 126].

There are more aspects of GIT involvement treatment. Regarding GERD, some studies reported favourable effect of GABA-B (gamma-aminobutyric acid receptor type B) agonists or metabotropic glutamate receptor antagonists (mGluR), which slow the decrease of basal LES pressure [127]. However, the beneficial effect has yet to be studied in SSc [86]. New pharmacological targets are still investigated, e.g. nitrous oxide synthase, cannabinoid, muscarinic or opioid receptors, etc., which reduce the transient LES relaxation. Surgical intervention is not generally recommended in SSc, because of association with increased risk of complications compared to general population, especially worsening of dysphagia [86].

Interventional endoscopy is the method of choice in indicated patients, e.g. endoscopic dilation of confirmed strictures should not be performed empirically due to the risk of perforation [128–130]. Laser or argon plasma coagulation is performed in GAVE, after adequate supplementation therapy of anaemia. Surgery should be the last solution after all strategies fail [86, 131].

Intestinal pseudo-obstruction requires exclusion of mechanical obstruction (RDG or computer tomography). Basal therapeutic approach lies in bowel rest, nutritional support, correcting electrolyte imbalance and use of prokinetics and antibiotics for coexisting SIBO [86]. In most cases (70%), this conservative treatment leads to spontaneous resolution. Some patients are indicated for surgery (9%) [132]. Subcutaneous octreotide at doses 50–200 micrograms per day is also recommended [86].

Treatment of large bowel symptoms is mainly symptomatic, including dietary measure and administration of laxatives or antidiarrhoeal drugs according to the dominant symptomatology [86]. Before the treatment of constipation, obstruction has to be excluded and current medication should be revised to avoid constipating drugs [133]. Aetiology of diarrhoea should be evaluated to exclude other aetiology, e.g. infections or other autoimmune disorders (celiac disease, microscopic colitis, amyloidosis). Antidiarrhoeal drugs (loperamide) have to be used with caution, because of the risk of pseudo-obstruction [86]. Bile acid sequestrants can be used to improve fat malabsorption in case of SIBO [133]. Incontinence is difficult to treat and requires complex approach consisting of management of diarrhoea, behavioural therapy (anorectal biofeedback), pelvic-floor exercise and eventually neuronal stimulation of sacral nerve—a microsurgery intervention [86].

8.2 Therapy of malnutrition

Enteral and sometimes long-term parenteral nutrition is often needed in progressive and advanced disease [1]. There are no studies available on enteral nutrition in SSc patients [83]. The North American expert panel recommends dietary supplementation in similar manner to treatment in patients with chronic diseases. In case of gastroparesis, dietary measures are recommended (low-fibre, low-fat, frequent small meals and higher content of liquid) along with regular monthly monitoring of body weight [83]. Alternative ways of enteral nutrition in case of insufficient oral alimentation are gastric or jejunal feeding [1]: percutaneous endoscopic gastrostomy (PEG) tube feeding, nasojejunal tube, or percutaneous or surgically placed enteral tube feeding in case of refractory gastroparesis and preserved normal small bowel function, or by PN [134, 135].

PN is an emerging option of treatment for patients with refractory malnutrition, where the EN is not sufficient (e.g. SIBO) or where surgical enteral nutrition may be difficult to provide (severe cutaneous fibrosis and thickening) [1]. The main disadvantages of PN are in general the cost and PN-related complications: catheter-related bloodstream infections; liver function abnormalities (e.g. cholestasis); metabolic bone disease; fluid overload, especially in patients with ILD and pulmonary arterial hypertension; electrolyte imbalances; and risk of central vein thrombosis in predisposed patients [136–140]. Moreover, specific problems with PN in SSc are caused by skin involvement, poor quality of veins due to vasculopathy and hand deformities requiring assistance with PN infusion [1].

Data on long-term PN in SSc patients are lacking. However, based on studies on PN in patients with chronic intestinal pathology and the data from retrospective studies on PN nutrition in SSc patients, which reported the improvement of quality of life and patients' profit from this therapy, this therapeutic approach is considered as effective in SSc patients [136, 141–144]. Regular monitoring for complications, control of body weight and adequate altering of nutrient supplements are recommended, along with the establishment of a team for patients' education, prevention of the catheter-related complications and optimising the nutrition intake. The optimal duration of PN needs to be determined [1].

8.3 Future therapeutic prospects

Novel therapeutic options of SSc GIT involvement are investigated, particularly immunosuppressive drugs targeting pro-fibrotic cytokines and IVIGs. Effect of IVIG therapy is multiple: anti-idiotypic-mediated neutralisation of muscarinic, anti-fibroblast or anti-endothelial cell circulating autoantibodies and reduction of pro-fibrotic cytokines. IVIG has a better safety profile compared to immunosuppressive drugs [14]. Observational studies confirmed its potential to improve GIT symptoms and reverse cholinergic dysfunction induced by M3-R autoantibodies in vivo [145–147]. Another therapeutic approach is targeting miRNA-29 by anti-miRNA chemically modified oligonucleotides [148]. However, future large-scale controlled studies are needed to confirm the beneficial effects of these promising approaches in SSc patients.

9. Conclusion

Gastrointestinal involvement is highly prevalent in systemic sclerosis, affects the majority of patients and can be hidden or can precede the obvious skin manifestation. Therefore, overall screening is recommended for early management of the

Field of research		To do
Aetiology	Genetic predisposition Infectious aetiology Environmental factors	Identify special haplotypes Identify pathoorganisms triggering the disease (e.g. *Helicobacter pylori* [9]) Identify the insult/toxin triggering the disease (smoking, exposition to toxic substances, etc.)
Pathogenesis Pathology	Autoantibodies Cytokines/chemokines	Association of well-known autoantibodies with the disease features and their role in pathogenesis (anti-topoisomerase I, anti-polymerase III, etc.) Identify new autoantibodies and their role in pathogenesis (e.g. IgG antibodies binding the M3 receptor for acetylcholine) Elucidate the role of cytokines/chemokines and cell immunity
Clinical features/ manifestation/phenotype	Onset of the disease Extent and severity of involvement Progression	Factors determining the course of the disease and clinical manifestation
Comorbidities	Malignancy Cardiovascular risk	Identify the factors/disease characteristics increasing the risk of malignancy Determine the risk compared to general population; identify the aetiology and type of specific manifestation
Nutrition Body composition	Markers of malnutrition Prevalence and character of negative changes of body composition	Composition of a sensitive and specific tool for evaluation of nutrition and complications leading to malnutrition (e.g. SIBO) Recommendation of an appropriate tool for examination of body composition and frequency of such testing
Therapy	Future specific therapy, targeted at specific mechanisms (molecules, antibodies, etc.) implicated in pathogenesis of the disease	IVIG (evidence of anti-idiotypic-mediated neutralisation of muscarinic, anti-fibroblast or anti-endothelial cell circulating autoantibodies and reduction of pro-fibrotic cytokines) Targeting RNA with small molecules; anti miRNA chemically modified oligonucleotides Conventional synthetic/targeted synthetic/ biologic/biosimilar DMARDs Stem-cell transplantation

Table 2.
Brief list of unmet needs and tasks for future research

gastrointestinal involvement until the ultimate damage develops. The pathophysiology and specific therapy are still the focus of research, with some promising prospects. To date, the cornerstone of the treatment is mainly symptomatic therapy and adequate nutritional support, best managed in cooperation with other specialists. The general impact of this involvement on patients' health status and quality of life should not be omitted. Large studies are required to examine aetiopathology and treatment options, including new therapeutic agents, and also complex impact of gastrointestinal involvement on patients' status (**Table 2**).

Acknowledgements

This chapter is supported by NV18-01-00161 A, MHCR 023728 and GAUK 312218.

Author details

Sabina Oreska and Michal Tomcik*
Institute of Rheumatology, Department of Rheumatology, Faculty of Medicine, Charles University, Prague, Czech Republic

*Address all correspondence to: tomcik@revma.cz

References

[1] Bharadwaj S, Tandon P, Gohel T, Corrigan ML, Coughlin KL, Shatnawei A, et al. Gastrointestinal manifestations, malnutrition, and role of enteral and parenteral nutrition in patients with Scleroderma. Journal of Clinical Gastroenterology. 2015;**49**(7):559-564

[2] LeRoy EC, Black C, Fleischmajer R, Jablonska S, Krieg T, Medsger TA Jr, et al. Scleroderma (systemic sclerosis): Classification, subsets and pathogenesis. The Journal of Rheumatology. 1988;**15**(2):202-205

[3] Sjogren RW. Gastrointestinal features of scleroderma. Current Opinion in Rheumatology. 1996;**8**(6):569-575

[4] Savarino E, Mei F, Parodi A, Ghio M, Furnari M, Gentile A, et al. Gastrointestinal motility disorder assessment in systemic sclerosis. Rheumatology (Oxford). 2013;**52**(6):1095-1100

[5] Steen VD, Medsger TA Jr. Severe organ involvement in systemic sclerosis with diffuse scleroderma. Arthritis and Rheumatism. 2000;**43**(11):2437-2444

[6] Sjogren RW. Gastrointestinal motility disorders in scleroderma. Arthritis and Rheumatism. 1994;**37**(9):1265-1282

[7] Bacher A, Mittoo S, Hudson M, Tatibouet S. Canadian Scleroderma Research G, Baron M. systemic sclerosis in Canada's north American native population: Assessment of clinical and serological manifestations. The Journal of Rheumatology. 2013;**40**(7):1121-1126

[8] Arnett FC, Howard RF, Tan F, Moulds JM, Bias WB, Durban E, et al. Increased prevalence of systemic sclerosis in a native American tribe in Oklahoma. Association with an Amerindian HLA haplotype. Arthritis and Rheumatism. 1996;**39**(8):1362-1370

[9] Radic M, Kaliterna DM, Bonacin D, Vergles JM, Radic J, Fabijanic D, et al. Is helicobacter pylori infection a risk factor for disease severity in systemic sclerosis? Rheumatology International. 2013;**33**(11):2943-2948

[10] Hudson M, Lo E, Lu Y, Hercz D, Baron M, Steele R, et al. Cigarette smoking in patients with systemic sclerosis. Arthritis and Rheumatism. 2011;**63**(1):230-238

[11] Bodukam V, Hays RD, Maranian P, Furst DE, Seibold JR, Impens A, et al. Association of gastrointestinal involvement and depressive symptoms in patients with systemic sclerosis. Rheumatology (Oxford). 2011;**50**(2):330-334

[12] Milette K, Hudson M, Korner A, Baron M, Thombs BD, Canadian Scleroderma Research G. Sleep disturbances in systemic sclerosis: Evidence for the role of gastrointestinal symptoms, pain and pruritus. Rheumatology (Oxford). 2013;**52**(9):1715-1720

[13] Omair MA, Lee P. Effect of gastrointestinal manifestations on quality of life in 87 consecutive patients with systemic sclerosis. The Journal of Rheumatology. 2012;**39**(5):992-996

[14] Kumar S, Singh J, Rattan S, DiMarino AJ, Cohen S, Jimenez SA. Review article: Pathogenesis and clinical manifestations of gastrointestinal involvement in systemic sclerosis. Alimentary Pharmacology & Therapeutics. 2017;**45**(7):883-898

[15] Gabrielli A, Avvedimento EV, Krieg T. Scleroderma. The New England Journal of Medicine. 2009;**360**(19):1989-2003

[16] Piasecki C, Chin J, Greenslade L, McIntyre N, Burroughs AK,

McCormick PA. Endoscopic detection of ischaemia with a new probe indicates low oxygenation of gastric epithelium in portal hypertensive gastropathy. Gut. 1995;**36**(5):654-656

[17] Malandrini A, Selvi E, Villanova M, Berti G, Sabadini L, Salvadori C, et al. Autonomic nervous system and smooth muscle cell involvement in systemic sclerosis: Ultrastructural study of 3 cases. The Journal of Rheumatology. 2000;**27**(5):1203-1206

[18] Russell ML, Friesen D, Henderson RD, Hanna WM. Ultrastructure of the esophagus in scleroderma. Arthritis and Rheumatism. 1982;**25**(9):1117-1123

[19] Kumar S, Singh J, Kedika R, Mendoza F, Jimenez SA, Blomain ES, et al. Role of muscarinic-3 receptor antibody in systemic sclerosis: Correlation with disease duration and effects of IVIG. American Journal of Physiology. Gastrointestinal and Liver Physiology. 2016;**310**(11):G1052-G1060

[20] Goldblatt F, Gordon TP, Waterman SA. Antibody-mediated gastrointestinal dysmotility in scleroderma. Gastroenterology. 2002;**123**(4):1144-1150

[21] Singh J, Mehendiratta V, Del Galdo F, Jimenez SA, Cohen S, DiMarino AJ, et al. Immunoglobulins from scleroderma patients inhibit the muscarinic receptor activation in internal anal sphincter smooth muscle cells. American Journal of Physiology. Gastrointestinal and Liver Physiology. 2009;**297**(6):G1206-G1213

[22] Singh J, Cohen S, Mehendiratta V, Mendoza F, Jimenez SA, Dimarino AJ, et al. Effects of scleroderma antibodies and pooled human immunoglobulin on anal sphincter and colonic smooth muscle function. Gastroenterology. 2012;**143**(5):1308-1318

[23] Cohen S, Fisher R, Lipshutz W, Turner R, Myers A, Schumacher R. The pathogenesis of esophageal dysfunction in scleroderma and Raynaud's disease. The Journal of Clinical Investigation. 1972;**51**(10):2663-2668

[24] Chizzolini C, Boin F. The role of the acquired immune response in systemic sclerosis. Seminars in Immunopathology. 2015;**37**(5):519-528

[25] O'Reilly S, Hugle T, van Laar JM. T cells in systemic sclerosis: A reappraisal. Rheumatology (Oxford). 2012;**51**(9):1540-1549

[26] Raja J, Denton CP. Cytokines in the immunopathology of systemic sclerosis. Seminars in Immunopathology. 2015;**37**(5):543-557

[27] Manetti M, Neumann E, Muller A, Schmeiser T, Saar P, Milia AF, et al. Endothelial/lymphocyte activation leads to prominent CD4+ T cell infiltration in the gastric mucosa of patients with systemic sclerosis. Arthritis and Rheumatism. 2008;**58**(9):2866-2873

[28] Manetti M, Neumann E, Milia AF, Tarner IH, Bechi P, Matucci-Cerinic M, et al. Severe fibrosis and increased expression of fibrogenic cytokines in the gastric wall of systemic sclerosis patients. Arthritis and Rheumatism. 2007;**56**(10):3442-3447

[29] Manetti M, Rosa I, Messerini L, Guiducci S, Matucci-Cerinic M, Ibba-Manneschi L. A loss of telocytes accompanies fibrosis of multiple organs in systemic sclerosis. Journal of Cellular and Molecular Medicine. 2014;**18**(2):253-262

[30] Stumpf M, Cao W, Klinge U, Klosterhalfen B, Kasperk R, Schumpelick V. Increased distribution of collagen type III and reduced expression of matrix metalloproteinase 1 in patients with diverticular disease.

International Journal of Colorectal Disease. 2001;**16**(5):271-275

[31] Parker MW, Rossi D, Peterson M, Smith K, Sikstrom K, White ES, et al. Fibrotic extracellular matrix activates a profibrotic positive feedback loop. The Journal of Clinical Investigation. 2014;**124**(4):1622-1635

[32] O'Reilly S. MicroRNAs in fibrosis: Opportunities and challenges. Arthritis Research & Therapy. 2016;**18**:11

[33] Peng WJ, Tao JH, Mei B, Chen B, Li BZ, Yang GJ, et al. MicroRNA-29: A potential therapeutic target for systemic sclerosis. Expert Opinion on Therapeutic Targets. 2012;**16**(9):875-879

[34] Maurer B, Stanczyk J, Jungel A, Akhmetshina A, Trenkmann M, Brock M, et al. MicroRNA-29, a key regulator of collagen expression in systemic sclerosis. Arthritis and Rheumatism. 2010;**62**(6):1733-1743

[35] Veale BJ, Jablonski RY, Frech TM, Pauling JD. Orofacial manifestations of systemic sclerosis. British Dental Journal. 2016;**221**(6):305-310

[36] Jung S, Martin T, Schmittbuhl M, Huck O. The spectrum of orofacial manifestations in systemic sclerosis: A challenging management. Oral Diseases. 2017;**23**(4):424-439

[37] Avouac J, Sordet C, Depinay C, Ardizonne M, Vacher-Lavenu MC, Sibilia J, et al. Systemic sclerosis-associated Sjogren's syndrome and relationship to the limited cutaneous subtype: Results of a prospective study of sicca syndrome in 133 consecutive patients. Arthritis and Rheumatism. 2006;**54**(7):2243-2249

[38] Auluck A, Pai KM, Shetty C, Shenoi SD. Mandibular resorption in progressive systemic sclerosis: A report of three cases. Dento Maxillo Facial Radiology. 2005;**34**(6):384-386

[39] Rajapakse CN, Bancewicz J, Jones CJ, Jayson MI. Pharyngo-oesophageal dysphagia in systemic sclerosis. Annals of the Rheumatic Diseases. 1981;**40**(6):612-614

[40] Kirby DF, Chatterjee S. Evaluation and management of gastrointestinal manifestations in scleroderma. Current Opinion in Rheumatology. 2014;**26**(6):621-629

[41] Derk CT, Rasheed M, Spiegel JR, Jimenez SA. Increased incidence of carcinoma of the tongue in patients with systemic sclerosis. The Journal of Rheumatology. 2005;**32**(4):637-641

[42] Ntoumazios SK, Voulgari PV, Potsis K, Koutis E, Tsifetaki N, Assimakopoulos DA. Esophageal involvement in scleroderma: Gastroesophageal reflux, the common problem. Seminars in Arthritis and Rheumatism. 2006;**36**(3):173-181

[43] Vischio J, Saeed F, Karimeddini M, Mubashir A, Feinn R, Caldito G, et al. Progression of esophageal dysmotility in systemic sclerosis. The Journal of Rheumatology. 2012;**39**(5):986-991

[44] Thonhofer R, Siegel C, Trummer M, Graninger W. Early endoscopy in systemic sclerosis without gastrointestinal symptoms. Rheumatology International. 2012;**32**(1):165-168

[45] Wipff J, Allanore Y, Soussi F, Terris B, Abitbol V, Raymond J, et al. Prevalence of Barrett's esophagus in systemic sclerosis. Arthritis and Rheumatism. 2005;**52**(9):2882-2888

[46] Wipff J, Coriat R, Masciocchi M, Caramaschi P, Derk CT, Hachulla E, et al. Outcomes of Barrett's oesophagus related to systemic sclerosis: A 3-year EULAR Scleroderma trials and Research prospective follow-up study. Rheumatology (Oxford). 2011;**50**(8):1440-1444

[47] Crowell MD, Umar SB, Griffing WL, DiBaise JK, Lacy BE, Vela MF. Esophageal motor abnormalities in patients with Scleroderma: Heterogeneity, risk factors, and effects on quality of life. Clinical Gastroenterology and Hepatology. 2017;**15**(2):207-13 e1

[48] Richardson C, Agrawal R, Lee J, Almagor O, Nelson R, Varga J, et al. Esophageal dilatation and interstitial lung disease in systemic sclerosis: A cross-sectional study. Seminars in Arthritis and Rheumatism. 2016;**46**(1):109-114

[49] American Thoracic Society. Idiopathic pulmonary fibrosis: diagnosis and treatment. International consensus statement. American Thoracic Society (ATS), and the European Respiratory Society (ERS). American Journal of Respiratory and Critical Care Medicine 2000;**161**(2 Pt 1):646-664

[50] Watson M, Hally RJ, McCue PA, Varga J, Jimenez SA. Gastric antral vascular ectasia (watermelon stomach) in patients with systemic sclerosis. Arthritis and Rheumatism. 1996;**39**(2):341-346

[51] Baron M, Hudson M, Steele R. Canadian Scleroderma Research G. malnutrition is common in systemic sclerosis: Results from the Canadian scleroderma research group database. The Journal of Rheumatology. 2009;**36**(12):2737-2743

[52] Marie I, Gourcerol G, Leroi AM, Menard JF, Levesque H, Ducrotte P. Delayed gastric emptying determined using the 13C-octanoic acid breath test in patients with systemic sclerosis. Arthritis and Rheumatism. 2012;**64**(7):2346-2355

[53] Marie I, Antonietti M, Houivet E, Hachulla E, Maunoury V, Bienvenu B, et al. Gastrointestinal mucosal abnormalities using videocapsule endoscopy in systemic sclerosis. Alimentary Pharmacology & Therapeutics. 2014;**40**(2):189-199

[54] Hung EW, Mayes MD, Sharif R, Assassi S, Machicao VI, Hosing C, et al. Gastric antral vascular ectasia and its clinical correlates in patients with early diffuse systemic sclerosis in the SCOT trial. The Journal of Rheumatology. 2013;**40**(4):455-460

[55] Marie I, Ducrotte P, Antonietti M, Herve S, Levesque H. Watermelon stomach in systemic sclerosis: Its incidence and management. Alimentary Pharmacology & Therapeutics. 2008;**28**(4):412-421

[56] Ingraham KM, O'Brien MS, Shenin M, Derk CT, Steen VD. Gastric antral vascular ectasia in systemic sclerosis: Demographics and disease predictors. The Journal of Rheumatology. 2010;**37**(3):603-607

[57] Ghrenassia E, Avouac J, Khanna D, Derk CT, Distler O, Suliman YA, et al. Prevalence, correlates and outcomes of gastric antral vascular ectasia in systemic sclerosis: A EUSTAR case-control study. The Journal of Rheumatology. 2014;**41**(1):99-105

[58] Lazzaroni MG, Cavazzana I, Colombo E, Dobrota R, Hernandez J, Hesselstrand R, et al. Malignancies in patients with anti-RNA polymerase III antibodies and systemic sclerosis: Analysis of the EULAR Scleroderma trials and Research cohort and possible recommendations for screening. The Journal of Rheumatology. 2017;**44**(5):639-647

[59] Gregersen H, Liao D, Pedersen J, Drewes AM. A new method for evaluation of intestinal muscle contraction properties: Studies in normal subjects and in patients with systemic sclerosis. Neurogastroenterology and Motility. 2007;**19**(1):11-19

[60] Valenzuela A, Li S, Becker L, Fernandez-Becker N, Khanna D, Nguyen L, et al. Intestinal pseudo-obstruction in patients with systemic sclerosis: An analysis of the Nationwide inpatient sample. Rheumatology (Oxford). 2016;**55**(4):654-658

[61] Marie I, Ducrotte P, Denis P, Menard JF, Levesque H. Small intestinal bacterial overgrowth in systemic sclerosis. Rheumatology (Oxford). 2009;**48**(10):1314-1319

[62] Abu-Shakra M, Guillemin F, Lee P. Gastrointestinal manifestations of systemic sclerosis. Seminars in Arthritis and Rheumatism. 1994;**24**(1):29-39

[63] Balbir-Gurman A, Brook OR, Chermesh I, Braun-Moscovici Y. Pneumatosis cystoides intestinalis in scleroderma-related conditions. Internal Medicine Journal. 2012;**42**(3):323-329

[64] Kaneko M, Sasaki S, Teruya S, Ozaki K, Ishimaru K, Terai E, et al. Pneumatosis Cystoides intestinalis in patients with systemic sclerosis: A case report and review of 39 Japanese cases. Case Reports in Gastrointestinal Medicine. 2016;**2016**:2474515

[65] Di Ciaula A, Covelli M, Berardino M, Wang DQ, Lapadula G, Palasciano G, et al. Gastrointestinal symptoms and motility disorders in patients with systemic scleroderma. BMC Gastroenterology. 2008;**8**:7

[66] Heyt GJ, Oh MK, Alemzadeh N, Rivera S, Jimenez SA, Rattan S, et al. Impaired rectoanal inhibitory response in scleroderma (systemic sclerosis): An association with fecal incontinence. Digestive Diseases and Sciences. 2004;**49**(6):1040-1045

[67] Trezza M, Krogh K, Egekvist H, Bjerring P, Laurberg S. Bowel problems in patients with systemic sclerosis. Scandinavian Journal of Gastroenterology. 1999;**34**(4):409-413

[68] Fynne L, Worsoe J, Laurberg S, Krogh K. Faecal incontinence in patients with systemic sclerosis: Is an impaired internal anal sphincter the only cause? Scandinavian Journal of Rheumatology. 2011;**40**(6):462-466

[69] Koh CE, Young CJ, Wright CM, Byrne CM, Young JM. The internal anal sphincter in systemic sclerosis. Diseases of the Colon and Rectum. 2009;**52**(2):315-318

[70] Riviere E, Vergniol J, Reffet A, Lippa N, Le Bail B, de Ledinghen V. Gastric variceal bleeding uncovering a rare association of CREST syndrome, primary biliary cirrhosis, nodular regenerative hyperplasia and pulmonary hypertension. European Journal of Gastroenterology & Hepatology. 2010;**22**(9):1145-1148

[71] Colina F, Pinedo F, Solis JA, Moreno D, Nevado M. Nodular regenerative hyperplasia of the liver in early histological stages of primary biliary cirrhosis. Gastroenterology. 1992;**102**(4 Pt 1):1319-1324

[72] Hartleb M, Gutkowski K, Milkiewicz P. Nodular regenerative hyperplasia: Evolving concepts on underdiagnosed cause of portal hypertension. World Journal of Gastroenterology. 2011;**17**(11):1400-1409

[73] Assassi S, Fritzler MJ, Arnett FC, Norman GL, Shah KR, Gourh P, et al. Primary biliary cirrhosis (PBC), PBC autoantibodies, and hepatic parameter abnormalities in a large population of systemic sclerosis patients. The Journal of Rheumatology. 2009;**36**(10):2250-2256

[74] Reynolds TB, Denison EK, Frankl HD, Lieberman FL, Peters RL. Primary biliary cirrhosis with scleroderma, Raynaud's phenomenon and telangiectasia. New Syndrome. American Journal of Medicine. 1971;**50**(3):302-312

[75] Cavazzana I, Ceribelli A, Taraborelli M, Fredi M, Norman G, Tincani A, et al. Primary biliary cirrhosis-related autoantibodies in a large cohort of Italian patients with systemic sclerosis. The Journal of Rheumatology. 2011;**38**(10):2180-2185

[76] Rigamonti C, Shand LM, Feudjo M, Bunn CC, Black CM, Denton CP, et al. Clinical features and prognosis of primary biliary cirrhosis associated with systemic sclerosis. Gut. 2006;**55**(3):388-394

[77] Assandri R, Monari M, Montanelli A. Development of systemic sclerosis in patients with autoimmune hepatitis: An emerging overlap syndrome. Gastroenterology and Hepatology from Bed to Bench. 2016;**9**(3):211-219

[78] You BC, Jeong SW, Jang JY, Goo SM, Kim SG, Kim YS, et al. Liver cirrhosis due to autoimmune hepatitis combined with systemic sclerosis. The Korean Journal of Gastroenterology. 2012;**59**(1):48-52

[79] Skare TL, Nisihara RM, Haider O, Azevedo PM, Utiyama SR. Liver autoantibodies in patients with scleroderma. Clinical Rheumatology. 2011;**30**(1):129-132

[80] Shawis TN, Chaloner C, Herrick AL, Jayson MI. Pancreatic function in systemic sclerosis. British Journal of Rheumatology. 1996;**35**(3):298-299

[81] Abraham AA, Joos A. Pancreatic necrosis in progressive systemic sclerosis. Annals of the Rheumatic Diseases. 1980;**39**(4):396-398

[82] Caporali R, Caccialanza R, Bonino C, Klersy C, Cereda E, Xoxi B, et al. Disease-related malnutrition in outpatients with systemic sclerosis. Clinical Nutrition. 2012;**31**(5):666-671

[83] Krause L, Becker MO, Brueckner CS, Bellinghausen CJ, Becker C, Schneider U, et al. Nutritional status as marker for disease activity and severity predicting mortality in patients with systemic sclerosis. Annals of the Rheumatic Diseases. 2010;**69**(11):1951-1957

[84] Baubet T, Ranque B, Taieb O, Berezne A, Bricou O, Mehallel S, et al. Mood and anxiety disorders in systemic sclerosis patients. Presse Médicale. 2011;**40**(2):e111-e119

[85] Baron M, Bernier P, Cote LF, Delegge MH, Falovitch G, Friedman G, et al. Screening and therapy for malnutrition and related gastro-intestinal disorders in systemic sclerosis: Recommendations of a north American expert panel. Clinical and Experimental Rheumatology. 2010;**28**(2 Suppl 58): S42-S46

[86] Nagaraja V, McMahan ZH, Getzug T, Khanna D. Management of gastrointestinal involvement in scleroderma. Current Treatment Options in Rheumatology. 2015;**1**(1):82-105

[87] Tanner SB, Moore CF Jr. A review of the use of dual-energy X-ray absorptiometry (DXA) in rheumatology. Open access Rheumatology : Research and Reviews. 2012;**4**:99-107

[88] Frediani B, Baldi F, Falsetti P, Acciai C, Filippou G, Spreafico A, et al. Bone mineral density in patients with systemic sclerosis. Annals of the Rheumatic Diseases. 2004;**63**(3):326-327

[89] Carbone L, Tylavsky F, Wan J, McKown K, Cheng S. Bone mineral density in scleroderma. Rheumatology (Oxford). 1999;**38**(4):371-372

[90] Corrado A, Colia R, Mele A, Di Bello V, Trotta A, Neve A, et al. Relationship between body mass composition, bone mineral density, skin fibrosis and 25(OH) vitamin D serum

levels in systemic sclerosis. PLoS One. 2015;**10**(9):e0137912

[91] Marighela TF, Genaro Pde S, Pinheiro MM, Szejnfeld VL, Kayser C. Risk factors for body composition abnormalities in systemic sclerosis. Clinical Rheumatology. 2013;**32**(7):1037-1044

[92] Rosato E, Gigante A, Gasperini ML, Molinaro I, Di Lazzaro GG, Afeltra A, et al. Nutritional status measured by BMI is impaired and correlates with left ventricular mass in patients with systemic sclerosis. Nutrition. 2014;**30**(2):204-209

[93] Caramaschi P, Biasi D, Caimmi C, Barausse G, Gatti D, Ferrari M, et al. Relationship between body composition and both cardiovascular risk factors and lung function in systemic sclerosis. Clinical Rheumatology. 2014;**33**(1):77-82

[94] Katz PO, Gerson LB, Vela MF. Guidelines for the diagnosis and management of gastroesophageal reflux disease. The American Journal of Gastroenterology. 2013;**108**(3):308-328. quiz 29

[95] Ebert EC. Esophageal disease in scleroderma. Journal of Clinical Gastroenterology. 2006;**40**(9):769-775

[96] Camilleri M, Parkman HP, Shafi MA, Abell TL, Gerson L. American College of G. clinical guideline: Management of gastroparesis. The American Journal of Gastroenterology. 2013;**108**(1):18-37. quiz 8

[97] Ghoshal UC, Srivastava D, Ghoshal U, Misra A. Breath tests in the diagnosis of small intestinal bacterial overgrowth in patients with irritable bowel syndrome in comparison with quantitative upper gut aspirate culture. European Journal of Gastroenterology & Hepatology. 2014;**26**(7):753-760

[98] Quigley EM. Small intestinal bacterial overgrowth: What it is and what it is not. Current Opinion in Gastroenterology. 2014;**30**(2):141-146

[99] Khanna D, Hays RD, Park GS, Braun-Moscovici Y, Mayes MD, McNearney TA, et al. Development of a preliminary scleroderma gastrointestinal tract 1.0 quality of life instrument. Arthritis and Rheumatism. 2007;**57**(7):1280-1286

[100] Khanna D, Hays RD, Maranian P, Seibold JR, Impens A, Mayes MD, et al. Reliability and validity of the University of California, Los Angeles Scleroderma clinical trial consortium gastrointestinal tract instrument. Arthritis and Rheumatism. 2009;**61**(9):1257-1263

[101] Spiegel BM, Hays RD, Bolus R, Melmed GY, Chang L, Whitman C, et al. Development of the NIH patient-reported outcomes measurement information system (PROMIS) gastrointestinal symptom scales. The American Journal of Gastroenterology. 2014;**109**(11):1804-1814

[102] Nagaraja V, Hays RD, Khanna PP, Spiegel BM, Chang L, Melmed GY, et al. Construct validity of the patient-reported outcomes measurement information system gastrointestinal symptom scales in systemic sclerosis. Arthritis Care Res (Hoboken). 2014;**66**(11):1725-1730

[103] Stratton RJ, Hackston A, Longmore D, Dixon R, Price S, Stroud M, et al. Malnutrition in hospital outpatients and inpatients: Prevalence, concurrent validity and ease of use of the 'malnutrition universal screening tool' ('MUST') for adults. The British Journal of Nutrition. 2004;**92**(5):799-808

[104] Murtaugh MA, Frech TM. Nutritional status and gastrointestinal symptoms in systemic sclerosis patients. Clinical Nutrition. 2013;**32**(1):130-135

[105] Khanna D, Nagaraja V, Gladue H, Chey W, Pimentel M, Frech T. Measuring response in the gastrointestinal tract in systemic sclerosis. Current Opinion in Rheumatology. 2013;**25**(6):700-706

[106] Harrison E, Herrick AL, McLaughlin JT, Lal S. Malnutrition in systemic sclerosis. Rheumatology (Oxford). 2012;**51**(10):1747-1756

[107] Soudah HC, Hasler WL, Owyang C. Effect of octreotide on intestinal motility and bacterial overgrowth in scleroderma. The New England Journal of Medicine. 1991;**325**(21):1461-1467

[108] Kowal-Bielecka O, Fransen J, Avouac J, Becker M, Kulak A, Allanore Y, et al. Update of EULAR recommendations for the treatment of systemic sclerosis. Annals of the Rheumatic Diseases. 2017;**76**(8):1327-1339

[109] Pakozdi A, Wilson H, Black CM, Denton CP. Does long term therapy with lansoprazole slow progression of oesophageal involvement in systemic sclerosis? Clinical and Experimental Rheumatology. 2009;**27**(3 Suppl 54):5-8

[110] Hendel L, Hage E, Hendel J, Stentoft P. Omeprazole in the long-term treatment of severe gastro-oesophageal reflux disease in patients with systemic sclerosis. Alimentary Pharmacology & Therapeutics. 1992;**6**(5):565-577

[111] Hendel L. Hydroxyproline in the oesophageal mucosa of patients with progressive systemic sclerosis during omeprazole-induced healing of reflux oesophagitis. Alimentary Pharmacology & Therapeutics. 1991;**5**(5):471-480

[112] Eusebi LH, Rabitti S, Artesiani ML, Gelli D, Montagnani M, Zagari RM, et al. Proton pump inhibitors: Risks of long-term use. Journal of Gastroenterology and Hepatology. 2017;**32**(7):1295-1302

[113] Rackoff A, Agrawal A, Hila A, Mainie I, Tutuian R, Castell DO. Histamine-2 receptor antagonists at night improve gastroesophageal reflux disease symptoms for patients on proton pump inhibitor therapy. Diseases of the Esophagus. 2005;**18**(6):370-373

[114] Fiorucci S, Distrutti E, Gerli R, Morelli A. Effect of erythromycin on gastric and gallbladder emptying and gastrointestinal symptoms in scleroderma patients is maintained medium term. The American Journal of Gastroenterology. 1994;**89**(4):550-555

[115] Verne GN, Eaker EY, Hardy E, Sninsky CA. Effect of octreotide and erythromycin on idiopathic and scleroderma-associated intestinal pseudoobstruction. Digestive Diseases and Sciences. 1995;**40**(9):1892-1901

[116] Nikou GC, Toumpanakis C, Katsiari C, Charalambopoulos D, Sfikakis PP. Treatment of small intestinal disease in systemic sclerosis with octreotide: A prospective study in seven patients. Journal of Clinical Rheumatology. 2007;**13**(3):119-123

[117] Wehrmann T, Caspary WF. Effect of cisapride on esophageal motility in healthy probands and patients with progressive systemic scleroderma. Klinische Wochenschrift. 1990;**68**(12):602-607

[118] Horowitz M, Maddern GJ, Maddox A, Wishart J, Chatterton BE, Shearman DJ. Effects of cisapride on gastric and esophageal emptying in progressive systemic sclerosis. Gastroenterology. 1987;**93**(2):311-315

[119] Kahan A, Chaussade S, Gaudric M, Freitag B, Amor B, Menkes CJ, et al. The effect of cisapride on gastro-oesophageal dysfunction in systemic sclerosis: A controlled manometric study. British Journal of Clinical Pharmacology. 1991;**31**(6):683-687

[120] Limburg AJ, Smit AJ, Kleibeuker JH. Effects of cisapride on the esophageal motor function of patients with progressive systemic sclerosis or mixed connective tissue disease. Digestion. 1991;**49**(3):156-160

[121] Wang SJ, La JL, Chen DY, Chen YH, Hsieh TY, Lin WY. Effects of cisapride on oesophageal transit of solids in patients with progressive systemic sclerosis. Clinical Rheumatology. 2002;**21**(1):43-45

[122] Quigley EM. Cisapride: What can we learn from the rise and fall of a prokinetic? Journal of Digestive Diseases. 2011;**12**(3):147-156

[123] Grace E, Shaw C, Whelan K, Andreyev HJ. Review article: Small intestinal bacterial overgrowth--prevalence, clinical features, current and developing diagnostic tests, and treatment. Alimentary Pharmacology & Therapeutics. 2013;**38**(7):674-688

[124] Parodi A, Sessarego M, Greco A, Bazzica M, Filaci G, Setti M, et al. Small intestinal bacterial overgrowth in patients suffering from scleroderma: Clinical effectiveness of its eradication. The American Journal of Gastroenterology. 2008;**103**(5):1257-1262

[125] Soifer LO, Peralta D, Dima G, Besasso H. Comparative clinical efficacy of a probiotic vs. an antibiotic in the treatment of patients with intestinal bacterial overgrowth and chronic abdominal functional distension: A pilot study. Acta Gastroenterologica Latinoamericana. 2010;**40**(4):323-327

[126] Frech TM, Khanna D, Maranian P, Frech EJ, Sawitzke AD, Murtaugh MA. Probiotics for the treatment of systemic sclerosis-associated gastrointestinal bloating/distention. Clinical and Experimental Rheumatology. 2011;**29**(2 Suppl 65): S22-S25

[127] Curcic J, Schwizer A, Kaufman E, Forras-Kaufman Z, Banerjee S, Pal A, et al. Effects of baclofen on the functional anatomy of the oesophago-gastric junction and proximal stomach in healthy volunteers and patients with GERD assessed by magnetic resonance imaging and high-resolution manometry: A randomised controlled double-blind study. Alimentary Pharmacology & Therapeutics. 2014;**40**(10):1230-1240

[128] Kaplan M, Mutlu EA, Jakate S, Bruninga K, Losurdo J, Losurdo J, et al. Endoscopy in eosinophilic esophagitis: "feline" esophagus and perforation risk. Clinical Gastroenterology and Hepatology. 2003;**1**(6):433-437

[129] Lew RJ, Kochman ML. A review of endoscopic methods of esophageal dilation. Journal of Clinical Gastroenterology. 2002;**35**(2):117-126

[130] Dubecz A, Stein HJ. Endoscopic versus surgical therapy for early cancer in Barrett's esophagus. Gastrointestinal Endoscopy. 2009;**70**(4):632-634

[131] Sebastian S, O'Morain CA, Buckley MJ. Review article: Current therapeutic options for gastric antral vascular ectasia. Alimentary Pharmacology & Therapeutics. 2003;**18**(2):157-165

[132] Mecoli C, Purohit S, Sandorfi N, Derk CT. Mortality, recurrence, and hospital course of patients with systemic sclerosis-related acute intestinal pseudo-obstruction. The Journal of Rheumatology. 2014;**41**(10):2049-2054

[133] Butt S, Emmanuel A. Systemic sclerosis and the gut. Expert Review of Gastroenterology & Hepatology. 2013;**7**(4):331-339

[134] Fynne L, Kruse A, Borre M, Sondergaard K, Krogh K. Percutaneous endoscopic gastrostomy in patients with systemic sclerosis. Scandinavian Journal of Rheumatology. 2010;**39**(3):266-268

[135] Keld R, Kinsey L, Athwal V, Lal S. Pathogenesis, investigation and dietary and medical management of gastroparesis. Journal of Human Nutrition and Dietetics. 2011;**24**(5):421-430

[136] Van Gossum A, Vahedi K, Abdel M, Staun M, Pertkiewicz M, Shaffer J, et al. Clinical, social and rehabilitation status of long-term home parenteral nutrition patients: Results of a European multicentre survey. Clinical Nutrition. 2001;**20**(3):205-210

[137] Lloyd DA, Vega R, Bassett P, Forbes A, Gabe SM. Survival and dependence on home parenteral nutrition: Experience over a 25-year period in a UK referral centre. Alimentary Pharmacology & Therapeutics. 2006;**24**(8):1231-1240

[138] Buchman AL, Iyer K, Fryer J. Parenteral nutrition-associated liver disease and the role for isolated intestine and intestine/liver transplantation. Hepatology. 2006;**43**(1):9-19

[139] Pironi L, Labate AM, Pertkiewicz M, Przedlacki J, Tjellesen L, Staun M, et al. Prevalence of bone disease in patients on home parenteral nutrition. Clinical Nutrition. 2002;**21**(4):289-296

[140] Puiggros C, Cuerda C, Virgili N, Chicharro ML, Martinez C, Garde C, et al. Catheter occlusion and venous thrombosis prevention and incidence in adult home parenteral nutrition (HPN) programme patients. Nutrición Hospitalaria. 2012;**27**(1):256-261

[141] Howard L. Home parenteral nutrition: Survival, cost, and quality of life. Gastroenterology. 2006;**130** (2 Suppl 1):S52-S59

[142] Ng SC, Clements PJ, Berquist WE, Furst DE, Paulus HE. Home central venous hyperalimentation in fifteen patients with severe scleroderma bowel disease. Arthritis and Rheumatism. 1989;**32**(2):212-216

[143] Grabowski G, Grant JP. Nutritional support in patients with systemic scleroderma. JPEN Journal of Parenteral and Enteral Nutrition. 1989;**13**(2):147-151

[144] Brown M, Teubner A, Shaffer J, Herrick AL. Home parenteral nutrition—An effective and safe long-term therapy for systemic sclerosis-related intestinal failure. Rheumatology (Oxford). 2008;**47**(2):176-179

[145] Poelman CL, Hummers LK, Wigley FM, Anderson C, Boin F, Shah AA. Intravenous immunoglobulin may be an effective therapy for refractory, active diffuse cutaneous systemic sclerosis. The Journal of Rheumatology. 2015;**42**(2):236-242

[146] Raja J, Nihtyanova SI, Murray CD, Denton CP, Ong VH. Sustained benefit from intravenous immunoglobulin therapy for gastrointestinal involvement in systemic sclerosis. Rheumatology (Oxford). 2016;**55**(1):115-119

[147] Clark KE, Etomi O, Denton CP, Ong VH, Murray CD. Intravenous immunoglobulin therapy for severe gastrointestinal involvement in systemic sclerosis. Clinical and Experimental Rheumatology. 2015;**33**(4 Suppl 91): S168-S170

[148] Ciechomska M, van Laar J, O'Reilly S. Current frontiers in systemic sclerosis pathogenesis. Experimental Dermatology. 2015;**24**(6):401-406

Chapter 4

Systemic Sclerosis Mimics

Ondřej Kodet and Sabína Oreská

Abstract

Many clinical conditions are presenting with sclerosis of the skin and with tissue fibrosis. These conditions may be confused with systemic sclerosis (SSc, scleroderma). These diseases and disabilities are generally referred to as systemic sclerosis mimics or scleroderma-like syndromes. These disorders have very different etiologies and often an unclear pathogenetic mechanism. Distinct clinical characteristics, skin histology, and disease associations may allow distinguishing these conditions from systemic sclerosis and from each other. A histopathological examination with clinicopathological correlation for diagnosis is important to spare the patients from ineffective treatments and inadequate management. In this chapter, we discussed localized scleroderma, lichen sclerosus, nephrogenic systemic fibrosis, eosinophilic fasciitis, scleromyxedema, and scleredema. These are often detected in the primary care setting and referred to rheumatologists for further evaluation. Rheumatologists, or preferably in collaboration with a dermatologist, must be able to promptly recognize them to provide valuable prognostic information and appropriate treatment options for affected patients.

Keywords: localized scleroderma, lichen sclerosus, eosinophilic fasciitis, nephrogenic systemic fibrosis, scleromyxedema, scleredema

1. Introduction

In this chapter, we discuss the groups of disorders classified as systemic sclerosis mimics. Localized and sometimes generalized skin stiffness is typical for this group of diseases. However, quite incongruous pathogenesis, underlying disease mechanisms and distinct organ involvement are significantly different in these conditions. This chapter describes the pathogenesis, clinical manifestation, histopathology findings, and therapeutic possibilities of the most common diseases that may cause difficulties in the differential diagnosis of systemic sclerosis.

2. Localized scleroderma, morphea

2.1 Introduction

Localized scleroderma is a clinically distinct inflammatory disease, primarily of the dermis and also subcutaneous fat [1]. The inflammation leads to scar-like sclerosis. Inflammatory infiltrates and changes of small vessels are similar in morphea and systemic sclerosis (SSc), but morphea has more asymmetric or linear skin localization and distribution than SSc, which has symmetrical distribution. Generalized morphea can prevent and mimic diffuse cutaneous SSc, but this clinical variant does not have Raynaud's phenomenon, digital sclerosis and lung, and gastrointestinal tract manifestation of the disease. Morphea is responsible for the morbidity of the patient such as skin tightness, joint mobility reduction leading to contractures, growth retardation, and pain [1–3].

2.2 Epidemiology

Morphea typically develops in adults, although morphea can occur at any age. The incidence of morphea is 3 per 100,000 people, and the prevalence of morphea increases with age. The mean age of disease onset is 45 years. Morphea is more prevalent in women than in men (2.6:1), except linear morphea, which has no gender preference [2–4].

2.3 Pathogenesis

The cause of the disease is unknown. Coexistence of various forms of scleroderma and the rare possibility of progression of localized scleroderma into SSc indicate that both types represent different manifestations of the same pathological process. Pathogenesis may be due to participation of environmental influences, immunological disorders, and infections, e.g., association with *Borrelia burgdorferi* [3]. Sclerosis of the skin is induced by vascular damage, activated T cells, and accented connective tissue production by dermal fibroblasts. Vascular changes represent a reduction in the number of capillaries. Enhanced production of collagen and other extracellular matrix proteins and components is induced by T-cell-derived cytokines, interleukin 4 (IL-4), IL-13, and transforming growth factor beta (TGF-β) [3, 5, 6].

2.4 Clinical features

Morphea can be divided into several clinical groups: plaque-type morphea, linear morphea, generalized morphea, deep morphea, nodular morphea, and guttate morphea. Patient with morphea does not have involvement of internal organs and Raynaud's phenomenon. Some patients may have involvement of muscles, tendons, and joints or neurological or ophthalmological symptoms which depend more likely on anatomical site, e.g., in a patient with linear morphea [2].

2.5 Plaque-type morphea, circumscribed morphea

Plaque-type morphea is the most common variant, characterized by a slightly elevated, edematous, erythematous, or violaceous and livid plaque with oval to round or centrifugal distribution (**Figure 1**). The developmental stage of the disease may influence the clinical features: (i) inflammatory, (ii) sclerotic, and (iii) atrophic [1, 2].

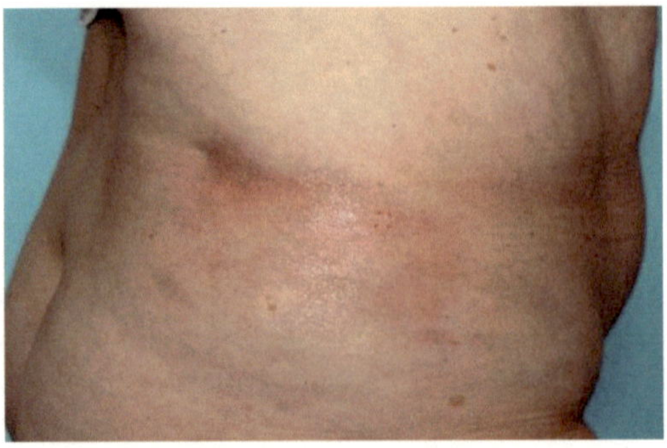

Figure 1.
Plaque-type morphea, lesion on the right side of the trunk. Plaques are surrounded by a dark red rim on the periphery with a yellowish white color center of the lesion as a result of the increasing deposition of connective tissue.

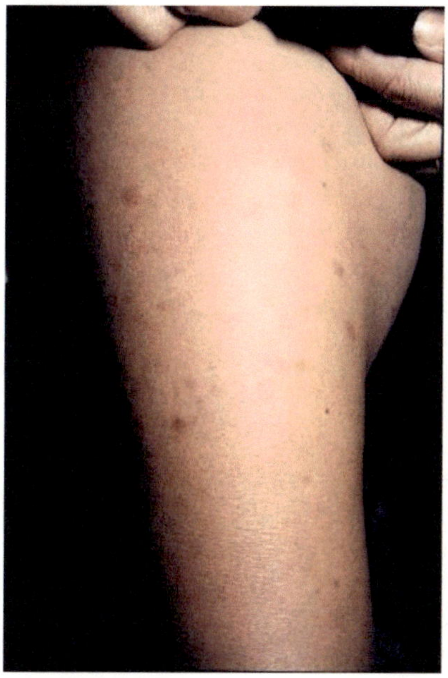

Figure 2.
Guttate morphea, multiple nummular lesions on the right thigh.

In the inflammatory phase, these are delimited striated skin plaques with the accentuated surface by skin pores, which resemble "orange peel" due to the edema of the corium expanding the follicular orifice. Plaques are surrounded by a violaceous rim on the periphery, indicating the active inflammatory stage of the disease. A yellowish-white color develops in the center of the lesion as a result of the increasing deposit of connective tissue [3]. In the sclerotic phase, the inflammatory border is absent. The skin of the lesion is smooth, shiny, and difficult or unable to be shaken. In the final (atrophic) phase, induration disappears; the plaques are soft, slightly sloping for skin and subcutaneous atrophy, and mostly gray-brown pigmented. Circumscribed morphea usually presents as single or multiple skin lesions. It is generally asymptomatic, but the central portion of the progressing lesion starts to get rigid and may be slightly painful [2, 3].

A different manifestation of morphea can be present. Guttate morphea presents as multiple rather superficial and nummular plaques (**Figure 2**).

Deep morphea represents sclerosis that affects the primarily deep parts of the dermis and subcutaneous fat (**Figure 3**).

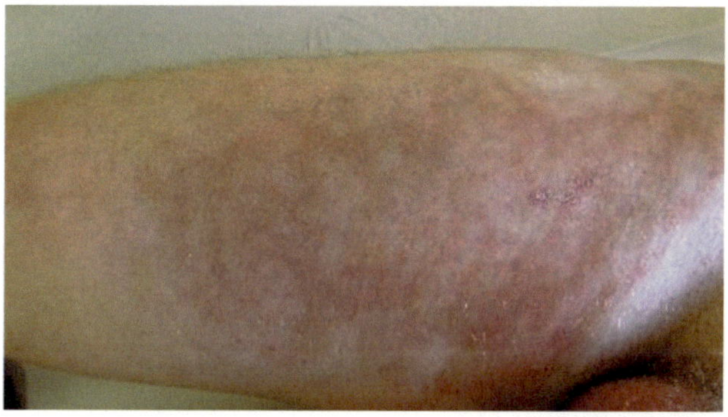

Figure 3.
Deep morphea, the affection of the front of the right thigh, mapping distribution of erythematous and whitish parts with visible scarring.

2.6 Linear morphea

Linear morphea is similar in the clinical feature to circumscribed morphea but with a linear distribution. Linear morphea initially starts as a linear erythematous streak or harmless lesion that later forms a scar-like band (**Figure 4**).

This scar-like band significantly impairs the mobility of the affected limb. Linear morphea can affect the underlying fascia, the muscle, and tendons. Linear morphea that transcends joints can significantly reduce movement and lead to developmental limb defects in children. Rarely, it can form bizarre configurations when copying Blaschko's lines [1, 3, 7].

2.7 "En coup de sabre"

The "en coup de sabre" represents a linear type of morphea of the head. This morphea is unilateral and extends from the forehead into the frontal scalp (**Figure 5**).

It usually starts as a small plaque with the surrounding inflammatory erythematous rim. Parry-Romberg syndrome is a rare variant of linear morphea of the forehead and scalp, with progressive loss of subcutaneous fat, with a smaller share of sclerosis [3, 8, 9].

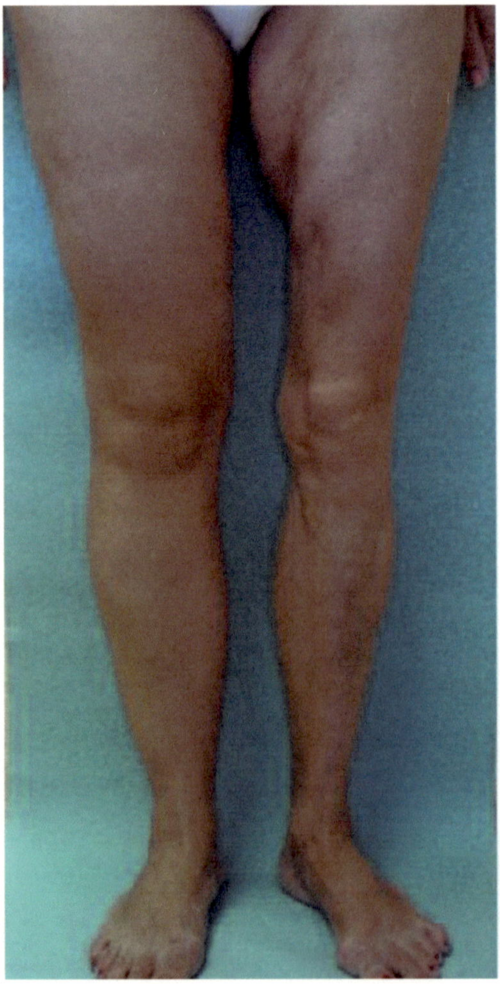

Figure 4.
Linear morphea, linear distribution of plaques, leading to atrophic changes in the affected limb.

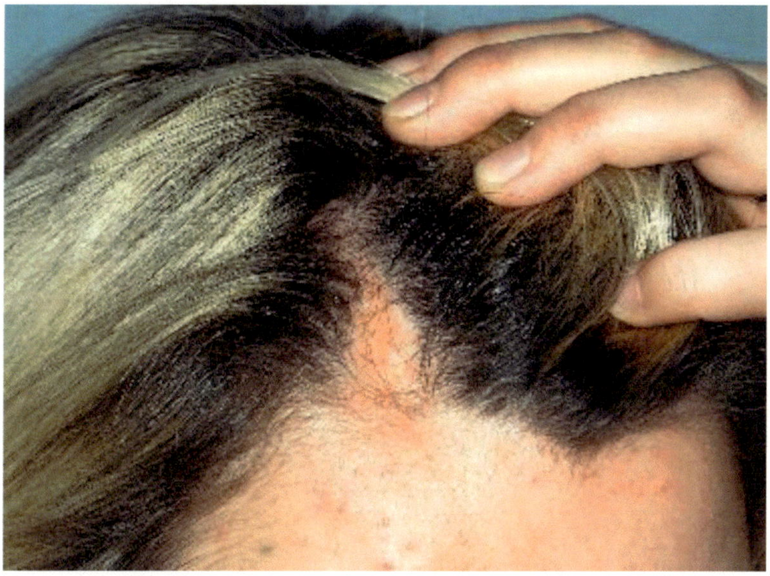

Figure 5.
"En coup de sabre" as linear morphea of the head. Linear scarring lesion on the forehead with an erythematous rim spreading to the scalp.

2.8 Generalized morphea

Generalized morphea begins as multiple plaque-type morphea on the trunk. This clinical variant is defined by the presence of ≥4 plaques involving at least two different anatomic sites (**Figure 6**).

In contrast to systemic sclerosis, generalized morphea does not present with sclerosis primarily involving acral skin or sclerodactyly, but this anatomical site can also be affected [10]. Apart from the skin, generalized morphea can also affect the subcutis and fascia, and be accompanied by slight changes in internal organs (especially the gastrointestinal tract and lungs) and the formation of joint contractures with mostly secondary joint involvement and movement limitation [11, 12]. Carapace-like tightening of the chest, can reduce breathing and cause swallowing difficulties.

2.9 Laboratory findings

Laboratory abnormalities are typically associated with generalized and linear morphea, but some patients with morphea have elevated antinuclear antibody (ANA). Reported rates of ANA positivity among patients with morphea range from 18 to 68%. Other autoantibodies that are detected less frequently than ANA in patients with morphea include anti-single-stranded DNA (ssDNA), anti-double-stranded DNA (dsDNA), antihistone, anti-topoisomerase IIα, antiphospholipid, and rheumatoid factor [1, 13].

2.10 Histopathology

The histopathological findings depend on the stage of the disease and area where the biopsy was taken (inflammatory border or central sclerotic lesion). Biopsy specimens for histology must include subcutaneous fat (**Figure 7**).

Biopsies performed from inflammatory lesions demonstrate an interstitial and perivascular inflammatory cell infiltrate composed primarily of $CD4^{+}$ T

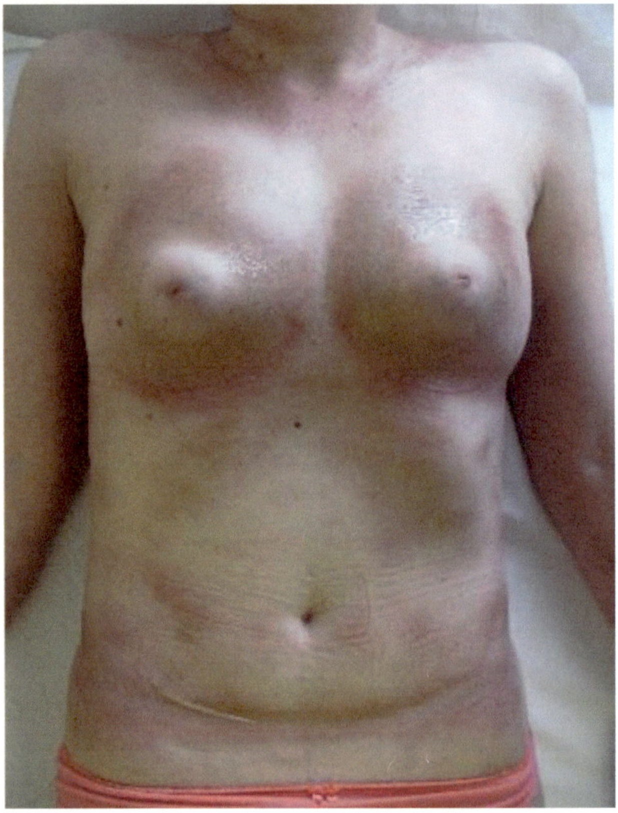

Figure 6.
Generalized morphea begins as multiple-plaque-type morphea on the abdomen, circularly affecting breasts and the neck. In the margins, lesions are with a rim of erythema, indicating the inflammatory stage of the disease.

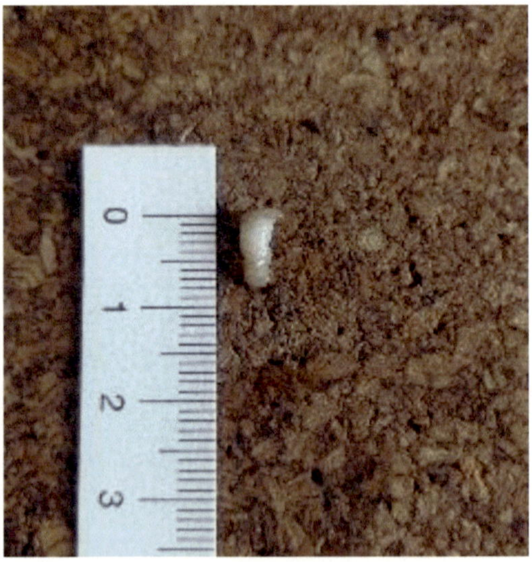

Figure 7.
Deep skin biopsy to subcutaneous fat after formaldehyde fixation.

cells, eosinophils, plasma cells, and mast cells. Inflammation may extend into the subcutaneous tissues. Furthermore, tissue edema, enlarged tortuous vessels, and thickened collagen bundles may be observed. Biopsy from a sclerotic lesion

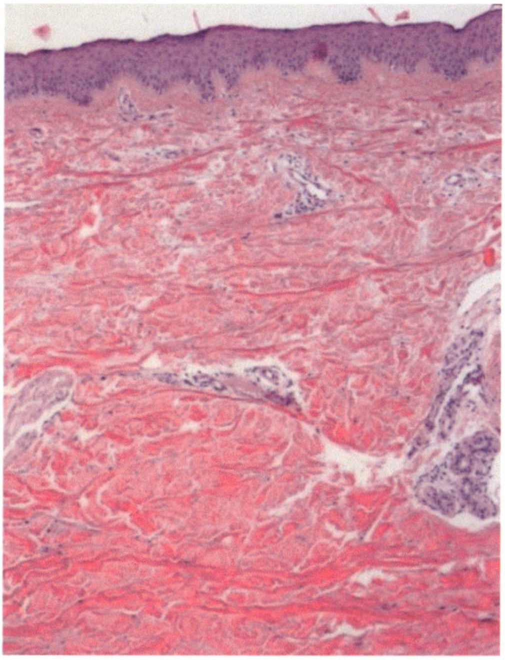

Figure 8.
Biopsy from a sclerotic lesion demonstrates homogenization of the papillary dermis and thickened collagen bundles extending into the reticular dermis.

demonstrates homogenization of the papillary dermis and thickened collagen bundles extending into the reticular dermis or beyond (**Figure 8**). In biopsy from deep morphea, the deep reticular dermis, subcutis, and fascia show sclerotic changes [14].

2.11 Differential diagnosis

A number of other disorders can present with clinical features that resemble morphea. Generalized morphea is necessary to distinguish from systemic sclerosis or scleredema diabeticorum. In addition to the skin sclerosis, systemic sclerosis generally begins with the Raynaud's phenomenon, and patients commonly exhibit initial puffiness and eventual sclerosis in the fingertips (sclerodactyly), usually accompanied by nail fold capillary changes. These changes are absent in patients with morphea. The differential diagnosis of plaque-type morphea includes lichen sclerosus, morpheaform basal cell carcinoma, and postirradiation morphea. Furthermore, we need to think of lipodermatosclerosis as fibrosing panniculitis with typical localization on the lower extremities or eosinophilic fasciitis. In some cases of limb involvement, pretibial myxedema or Lyme disease (acrodermatitis atrophicans) must be excluded [1, 13, 14].

2.12 Treatment

A variety of treatment options are available for patients with active lesions of morphea; however, evidence in support and success of these therapeutics modalities is limited. The expected outcome of successful therapy for morphea is not a complete healing or normal skin texture. In patients with progressive disease, successful treatment presents stopping the formation of new lesions and limiting the spreading of the disease [1, 15].

2.13 Topical and intralesional treatment

Topical therapies are unlikely to be effective for the disease involving the subcutis or deeper tissues and are not useful for preventing the development of new lesions in patients with rapidly progressive disease. Topical tacrolimus as tacrolimus 0.1% ointment may be effective for active, inflammatory morphea [16]. High potency topical and intralesional corticosteroids are widely used for the treatment of morphea; however, no formal studies have documented their efficacy. Topical vitamin D—vitamin D as topical calcipotriene 0.005% ointment—may inhibit effects on fibroblast proliferation, collagen synthesis, and T-cell activation. In some clinical studies, an improvement on this therapy was noted in limited numbers of patients [15, 17].

Imiquimod is a topical immunomodulator that induces interferon-gamma, a cytokine that inhibits TGF-beta and the production of extracellular matrix proteins. Imiquimod also downregulates the profibrotic cytokine IL-4. Limited data suggest that imiquimod is effective in some patients with plaque-type morphea [18].

It is possible to use phototherapy in patients with sclerotic diseases like morphea. Longer wavelengths of light as ultraviolet A (UVA) (320–400 nm) are capable of greater depth of penetration into the skin, and most studies of UV phototherapy in sclerotic skin disease have focused on the use of UVA light (320–400 nm). Fewer data are available on the use of PUVA therapy (a combination of UVA and topical or oral use of psoralens) and ultraviolet B (UVB) light (290–320 nm). Phototherapy is unlikely to be effective for morphea with deep involvement (subcutis, fascia, or muscle) and should not be considered as primary therapy alone [19].

2.14 Systemic treatment

Patients with the progressive disease require systemic therapy with methotrexate or corticosteroids. Methotrexate is the most appropriate systemic therapy for morphea. In patients with acute generalized or rapidly progressive disease, we combine treatment with systemic corticosteroids. Methotrexate is typically given for at least 6–12 months with a weekly dose of 15–25 mg. The systemic corticosteroids are usually tapered and discontinued after 3–4 months or pulse intravenous therapy is used instead (500–1000 mg of intravenous methylprednisolone sodium succinate for 3 consecutive days/month) [15, 20].

3. Morpheaform inflammatory syndromes/conditions

Some diseases and disorders with acrosclerosis and Raynaud's phenomenon have a clinical presentation similar to localized scleroderma. The etiology of these disorders is diverse and includes, e.g., secondary sclerosis after exposition to bleomycin, vinyl chloride, L-tryptophan, or toxic oils. Sclerosis can also be induced by endogenous metabolites, by x-irradiation, or during chronic graft-versus-host disease (GVHD) (**Figure 9**). Morphea-like lesion, eosinophilic fasciitis, and lichen sclerosus can also be observed in these patients [21].

3.1 Lipodermatosclerosis

3.1.1 Introduction

Typical changes associated with chronic venous insufficiency include erythema, induration, and hemosiderin pigmentary changes. But a variety of clinical

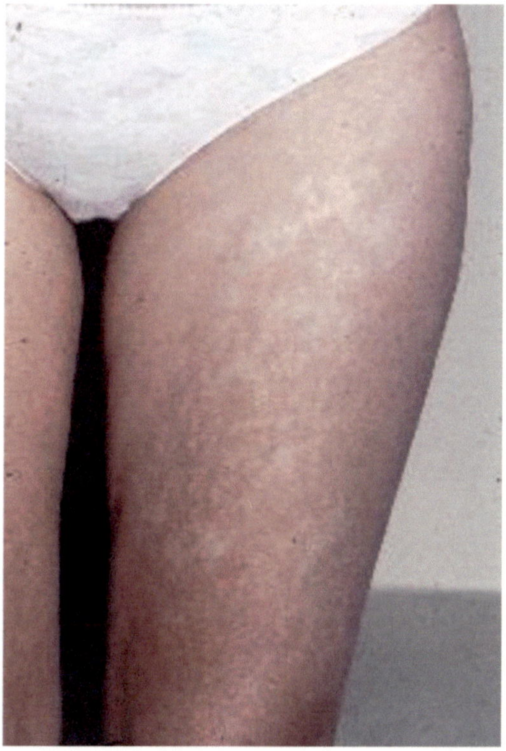

Figure 9.
Morphea-like lesion in a patient with GVHD. Post-inflammatory hyperpigmentation with whitish areas of sclerotic skin affecting the left thigh.

appearances and histopathologic findings also include sclerosis, or sclerosing panniculitis. The various manifestations of this panniculitis have been consolidated under the heading of lipodermatosclerosis or sclerosing panniculitis [22].

Lipodermatosclerosis typically manifests in patients, usually in women over the age of 40 years with chronic venous insufficiency as a result of chronic hypoxia. Venous hypertension leads to a compromised ability to reduce foot vein pressure during exercise. This change results in increased capillary permeability, with leakage of fibrinogen, with subsequent polymerization leading to formation of fibrin plaques around vessels. There may also be an abnormal regulation of angiogenesis in a patient with lipodermatosclerosis. For example, increased expression of vascular endothelial growth factor receptor 1 (VEGFR-1) can be a result of VEGF-mediated angiogenesis. Another factors may include local stimulation of collagen and obesity [23, 24].

3.1.2 Clinical features

Sclerosis affects the acral parts of the lower limbs symmetrically. The acute and progressive phase of lipodermatosclerosis presents with pain, erythema, and the formation of induration on the affected area of lower limbs. In the chronic phase, sclerosis of the dermis and subcutis is typically present, and sclerosis results in induration that is more sharply demarcated from the adjacent normal skin (**Figure 10**). Other gravity dependent sites such as the lower aspect of the abdominal pannus can also develop lipodermatosclerosis. At this point, the changes are relatively diffuse. Hyperpigmentation due to hemosiderin deposition or chronic ulceration of the lower limbs may also be present [22].

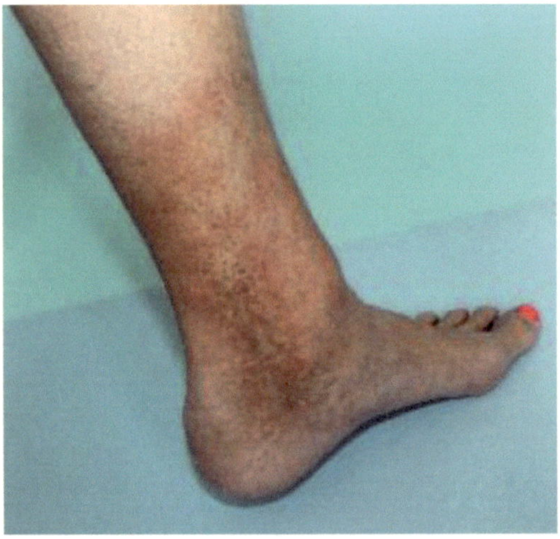

Figure 10.
Lipodermatosclerosis in a patient with chronic venous insufficiency. In this case erythema and sclerotic whitish induration on the medial part of the shank with the border of hemosiderin pigmentary changes are present.

3.1.3 Histopathology

Early lesions show mid-lobular panniculitis, a lymphocytic infiltrate in the septa, variable degrees of capillary congestion, and extravasation of erythrocytes with hemosiderin deposition. Chronic lesions show septal sclerosis and membranocytic change with a marked reduction in inflammation or lymphocytic infiltrate [25, 26].

3.1.4 Differential diagnosis

In differential diagnosis, it is necessary to distinguish inflammatory changes such as cellulitis and erysipelas but also erythema nodosum or erythema induratum. As induration develops and progresses, differentiation from morphea and scleromyxedema may be necessary. In morphea, subcutaneous involvement is predominantly septal, and lipophagic and lipodystrophic changes are not typically present [22, 25].

3.1.5 Treatment

Leg elevation and consistent compression therapy are crucial for the treatment of lipodermatosclerosis. Traditional anti-inflammatory therapies are usually ineffective, but topical or intralesional corticosteroids (e.g., triamcinolone 5–10 mg/cc) may bring relief and improvement with compression therapy [27].

3.2 Injection of vitamin K

Oil-soluble injection of vitamin K may be responsible for the eosinophilic reaction of the deep part of the dermis and subcutaneous fat, which may resemble localized eosinophilic fasciitis with similar clinical manifestation as deep morphea. This inflammation can result in dermal and subcutaneous atrophy [28].

3.3 Vaccination-associated morphea

Circumscribed morphea and deep morphea have been described after intramuscular injections of different types of vaccines. The etiology and antigens responsible for this type of inflammation have not been reliably elucidated [29].

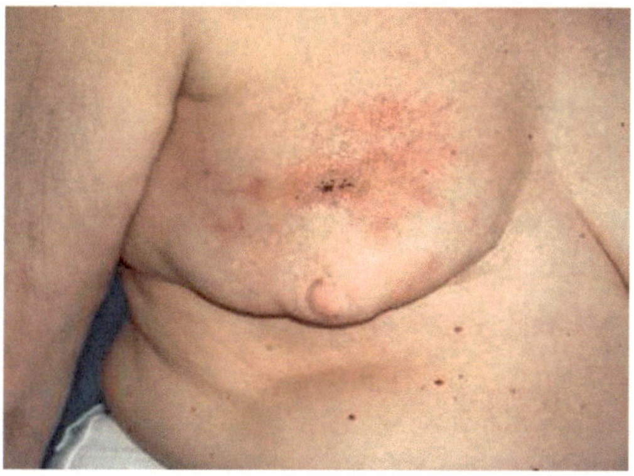

Figure 11.
Morphea-like lesion in a patient after x-irradiation for breast carcinoma. The erythematous and sclerodermic lesion on the right breast.

3.4 Paraffin and silicone injections or silicone implants

The leak of silicone from implants and silicone or paraffin injection after reconstructive or plastic surgery induce chronic inflammation that results in localized morphea-like lesion. The contribution to the induction of SSc, eosinophilic fasciitis, or mixed connective tissue disease has also been discussed [30].

3.5 Porphyrias

Porphyria cutanea tarda can lead to a morphea-like lesion and scarring in the chronic sun (UV)-exposed sites, such as the face, scalp, dorsal part of the hands, and upper part of the chest [31].

3.6 Radiation-induced morphea

X-Irradiation can induce sclerotic, chronic erythematous, and secondary pigmented lesions typically in a patient after irradiation of the chest and axillary region for breast carcinoma (**Figure 11**). The morphea-like lesions can start several years after radiation [32].

3.7 Differential diagnosis

The differential diagnosis is summarized in this paragraph, but the most important entity in the differential diagnosis of SSc or localized scleroderma is lichen sclerosus et atrophicus and scleromyxedema. Absence of overall symptoms and organ involvement is crucial [21].

4. Lichen sclerosus

Lichen sclerosus et atrophicus is an inflammatory disease, primarily of the superficial dermis or mucosa, which leads to white scar-like atrophy. Extragenital lichen sclerosus may itch and be cosmetically annoying. Genital lichen sclerosus causes dryness and persistent pruritus. Genital lichen leads to progressive atrophy, and functional impairment, which significantly reduces the quality of life.

4.1 Epidemiology

Prevalence of lichen sclerosus is unknown. This chronic disease occurs at all ages with a similar incidence in all races. The ratio of occurrence in men and women varies considerably, but in both sexes, the most affected area is the anogenital region (about 85% of patients, in women usually as a vulvar disease) [33, 34].

4.2 Pathogenesis

Association with the MHC class II antigen HLA-DQ7 was observed, but the specific genetic predisposition is unknown. Unspecific inflammation seems to be essential for the initiation and also the progression of lichen sclerosus. Autoantibodies such as those against the extracellular matrix protein 1 (ECM-1) were found in 80% of patients with lichen sclerosus. Moreover, in female patients with lichen sclerosus, there is a higher prevalence of autoimmune diseases (especially autoimmune thyroid disease) and ANA positivity than in male patients with lichen sclerosus [34–36].

4.3 Clinical features

Lichen sclerosus manifests by polygonal, bluish-white, shiny, slightly elevated maculopapules with a pointed follicular bounds of hyperkeratoses, which may be solitary or in groups. This skin lesion can be bounded with an area of erythema. The solitary lesion enlarges to plaques and to the scar-like lesion with a rough surface and skin atrophy (**Figure 12**).

More rarely, blistering with possible hemorrhagic content can be present (**Figure 13**). Extragenital predilection sites include supraclavicular localization, under the breasts, cubit, groin, loose wrist, and cross. Symptoms of extragenital lichen sclerosus are dryness and pruritus.

However, lichen sclerosus most frequently affects the anogenital region. In women, it typically affects the vulva and the perianal localization in figure-of-eight configuration (**Figure 14**). Genital lichen sclerosus begins as slightly elevated lesion of erythema, sometimes with erosions. During the chronic stage of the disease, the skin becomes shiny, sclerotic, and also hypopigmented. The scarring may affect the clitoris and labia, and disability may be significant or even make the sexual intercourse impossible. Although the disease may be symptom-free, it frequently causes severe pruritus and pain is a typical symptom. Another symptom may be dysuria or pain upon defecation [34, 37].

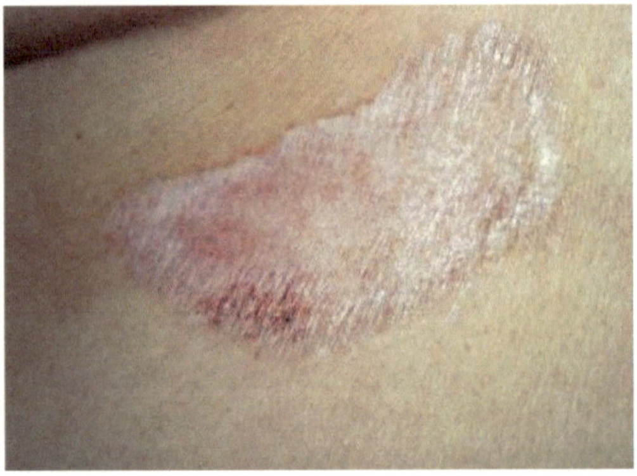

Figure 12.
Extragenital lichen sclerosus, slightly elevated plaque with scar-like presentation, with a whitish erythematous rim and skin atrophy.

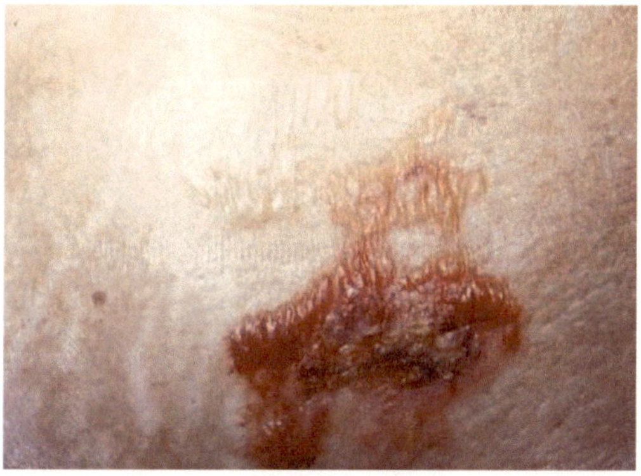

Figure 13.
Extragenital lichen sclerosus, whitish plaque with blisters and crusts. Blisters resemble hemorrhagic-like content.

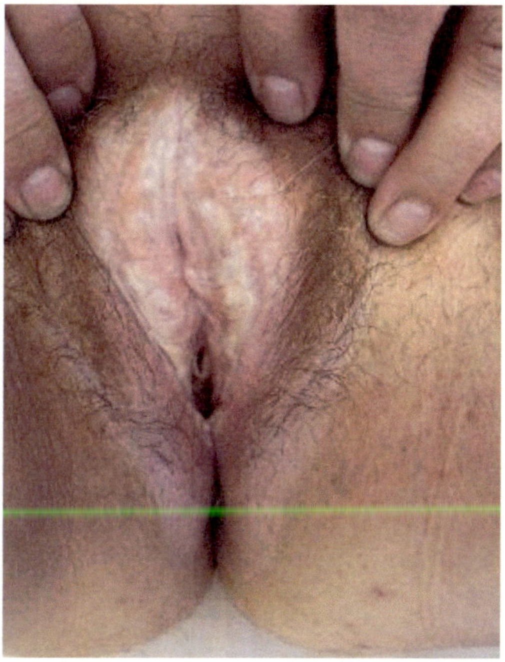

Figure 14.
Genital lichen sclerosus affects the labia minora, clitoris, and vulval vestibule. Whitish and erythematous plaques are also present in the labia majora, the perineum, and the perianal region.

4.4 Histopathology

Lichen sclerosus has a specific histopathological pattern. Initially, superficial dermal edema is associated with a band-like lymphocytic infiltrate. The epidermis is thinned and atrophic, with orthohyperkeratosis and vacuolar degeneration of the basal layer. Hyperkeratosis is especially pronounced at follicular openings and may lead to plugging. Vacuolar degeneration of the basal layer and flattening of the rete ridges predispose to the development of blisters, which may become hemorrhagic. The most important changes are found in the superficial dermis with the presence of homogenized collagen (**Figure 15**). Loss of elastic fibers is typical for lichen sclerosus and is not observed in morphea [38–40].

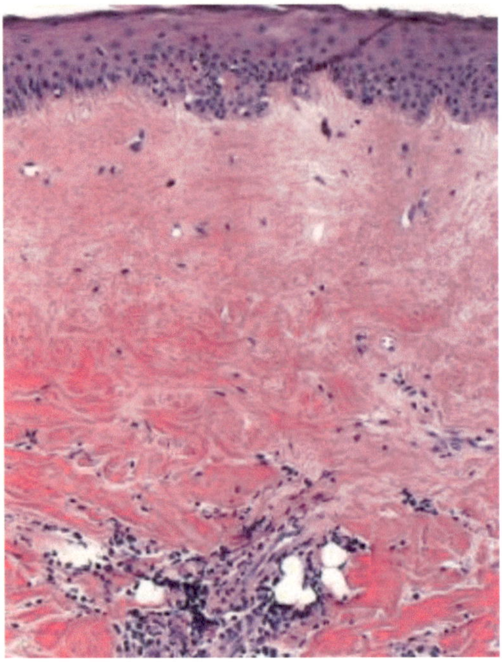

Figure 15.
Skin biopsy of extragenital lichen sclerosus where atrophic thinned epidermis and mild vacuolar degeneration of the basal layer are present. In the superficial dermis, homogenized collagen with perivascular lymphocytic infiltrates can be found.

4.5 Differential diagnosis

The differential diagnosis of extragenital lichen sclerosus includes morphea, vitiligo, tinea versicolor, anetoderma, or cutaneous lymphoma. In the case of genital lichen sclerosus, erosive lichen planus and erythroplasia of Queyrat must be considered.

Sometimes it is not possible to distinguish morphea from lichen because clinical and especially histopathological findings of both diseases can also be present in one patient or one biopsy [34].

4.6 Treatment

Topical medications, phototherapy, and systemic therapy have been used for the treatment of lichen sclerosus. The effect of topical corticosteroids was reported especially in genital lichen sclerosus, but mitigation has also been demonstrated in extragenital lichen. Effect of topical corticosteroid therapy has been reported in randomized treatment and retrospective studies. Phototherapy is preferred second-line treatment for patients with limited disease that cannot be effectively treated with topical corticosteroids. An alternative to topical corticosteroids is the use of calcineurin inhibitors pimecrolimus and tacrolimus despite concerns of possible increase of development of squamous cell carcinoma or reactivation of HPV [15, 37, 41].

The use of systemic therapy is limited to a small group of patients with progressive worsening of extragenital lichen sclerosus that failed to respond to a potent topical corticosteroid and phototherapy. For systemic therapy, methotrexate (15–20 mg/week) and systemic corticosteroids (1 g of intravenous methylprednisolone sodium succinate for 3 consecutive days/month) can be used [42].

5. Eosinophilic fasciitis

Eosinophilic fasciitis is a relatively recently described disease, characterized by fibrosing induration of the extremities and peripheral eosinophilia. In many patients strenuous physical activity precedes the development of this condition.

5.1 Clinical feature

Initial clinical manifestation includes painful edema of the extremities, which progresses to fibrosis and pseudo-inflammatory appearance (**Figure 16**). The manifestation of the disease is typically symmetrical on extremities without involvement of the hands, feet, and face [43].

Laboratory findings include elevation of ESR, hypergammaglobulinemia and peripheral eosinophilia which can be present in the early phase of the disease. ANA titer and complement level are usually normal. Pancytopenia, anemia, thrombocytopenia, myeloproliferative disorders, and monoclonal gammopathy have been reported in association with eosinophilic fasciitis. The diagnosis of eosinophilic fasciitis is established via fascial biopsy and/or by MRI [44].

5.2 Histopathology

Histologically eosinophils and mast cells are present, and dermal fibrosis with patchy infiltrates composed of lymphocytes and plasma cells are also present. In deep biopsy thickening of the fascia is typical, which may be 10–50 times the normal width [44].

5.3 Treatment

Once the diagnosis of eosinophilic fasciitis is established via fascial biopsy and/or MRI, prompt treatment is essential to preserve mobility and function and prevent joint contractures. Prompt therapy with oral corticosteroids (e.g., prednisone 1–2 mg/kg daily) is usually necessary for reduction or cessation of rapid disease progression and as prevention of mobility reduction and development of joint contractures. The response is typically noted within the first few weeks, and clinical improvement may be seen over several months. Alternatively, hydroxychloroquine, cyclosporine, dapsone, methotrexate, PUVA, or infliximab may be used alone or in combination with prednisone. Phototherapy as UVA1 can also be beneficial [45].

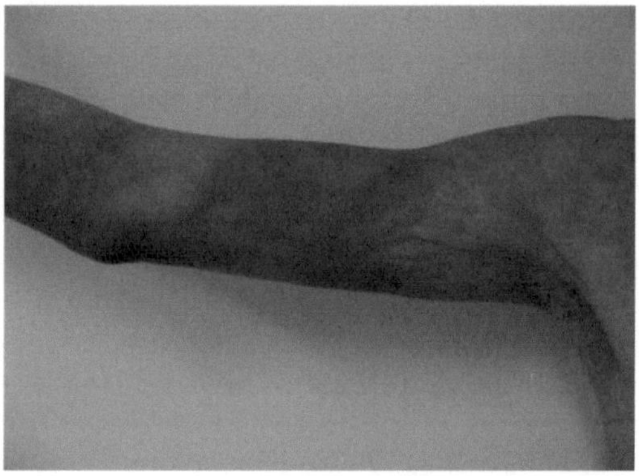

Figure 16.
Eosinophilic fasciitis with initial clinical manifestation of progressive fibrotic changes with pseudo-inflammatory appearance.

6. Nephrogenic systemic fibrosis

Nephrogenic systemic fibrosis is most often observed in middle-aged adults but has also been described in children and elderly patients. There is no gender or race predilection. Renal dysfunction and exposure to gadolinium-based contrast medium play a crucial role in the pathogenesis. Although the context use of the gadolinium in a patient with renal dysfunction is irrefutable, the mechanisms of fibrosis are still unknown [46, 47].

6.1 Clinical features

This disorder presents with large and thick, indurated plaques distributed symmetrically on the extremities and trunk. The skin lesions are irregular and erythematous with a tendency to develop hyperpigmentation. The manifestation on the extremities often results in joint contractures. The condition is frequently associated with considerable pain and loss of mobility. Extracutaneous manifestations include yellow scleral plaques and systemic fibrosis with involvement of the heart, lungs, and also skeletal muscles [48, 49].

6.2 Histopathology

A deep biopsy is necessary for diagnosis. Histologic features include increased dermal fibroblast-like cells with positivity for CD34 and procollagen I. Haphazard arrangement of thickened collagen bundles is also present. Furthermore, vascular proliferation and mucin deposition may also be present.

6.3 Treatment

Nephrogenic systemic fibrosis is refractory to treatment with corticosteroids and other immunosuppressive drugs. There have only been case reports of improvement with imatinib, rapamycin, phototherapy UVA1, PUVA, or plasmapheresis. Improvement in renal function after renal transplantation may improve this type of fibrosis [49].

7. Stiff skin syndrome

This dysfunction may be hereditary as a congenital disorder or acquired during early childhood. Familiar hereditary subtype is caused by heterozygosity for a mutation in the gene that encodes fibrillin-1 (FBN1). Dysfunction of this gene results in the production of giant collagen fibrils in the affected fascia [50].

7.1 Clinical features

Stiff skin syndrome is characterized by "rock hard" induration and thickening of the skin and subcutaneous tissues. Typical manifestation is on the buttocks and thighs with mild hypertrichosis without affecting the inguinal folds. This disorder does not affect the hands and feet. The condition is stable or slowly progressive, and abnormalities of internal organs are not typically observed. In differential diagnosis the disease may resemble scleredema, deep morphea, or linear scleroderma [51].

7.2 Histopathology

Histologically, significant thickness of fascia with deposition of hyaline without an associated inflammatory infiltrate can be found. Thickened collagen bundles and mucin deposition may be present in the dermis. The epidermis and papillary dermis are mostly without any pathologies [52].

7.3 Treatment

Treatment of stiff skin syndrome is very difficult, and no effective treatments have been reported. Physical therapy and regimen measures for the patient can help to prevent progressive joint contractures and immobility [51, 52].

8. Scleromyxedema

Scleromyxedema is a chronic idiopathic disorder characterized by papules and lesion of induration with dermal mucin deposition and with an increase of dermal collagen resulting in skin sclerosis. Many patients with scleromyxedema have monoclonal gammopathy, with systemic or lethal manifestations. Scleromyxedema represents a generalized variant that needs to be distinguished from localized lichen myxedematosus (variant without sclerosis and paraproteinemia) [53].

8.1 Pathogenesis

The exact pathogenesis of scleromyxedema is unknown, typically affecting middle-aged adults of both sexes equally. The role of the associated monoclonal gammopathy remains a matter of debate, because, for example, paraprotein levels do not correlate with progression of the disease. But clinical remission of scleromyxedema, during the reduction of paraprotein, that follows after autologous hematopoietic stem cell transplantation was described [53, 54].

8.2 Clinical features

In the clinical manifestation of scleromyxedema, typically widespread and symmetrically firm, waxy, and closely aligned papules are present (**Figure 17**).

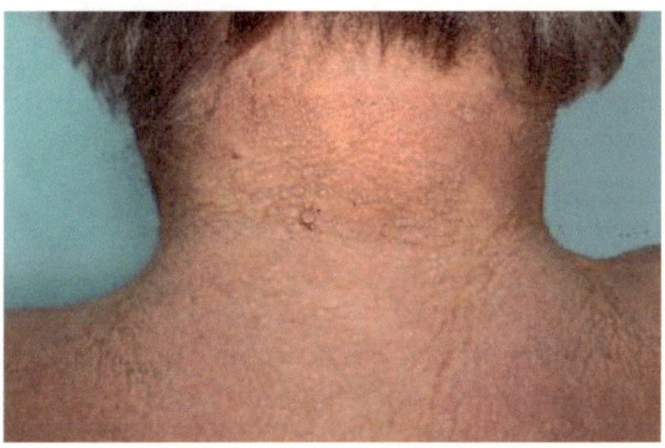

Figure 17.
Scleromyxedema. Numerous skin-colored papules of the neck.

Predilection localizations include the head and neck, upper trunk, forearms, and thighs and the proximal parts of fingers. The surrounding skin is shiny with sclerodermoid appearance. Deep longitudinal furrowing is typically involved on the glabella. Strong and rigid infiltrates of the face can result in the face of a lionlike face. As the condition progresses, erythematous and infiltrated plaques may be present with skin stiffening, sclerodactyly, and decreased motility of the mouth and joints.

Scleromyxedema is almost always associated with paraproteinemia. The monoclonal gammopathy is usually IgG and the light chains are more commonly lambda. Patients with scleromyxedema can have a number of internal manifestations, such as dysphagia, proximal muscle weakness due to myositis, peripheral neuropathy, arthropathies, carpal tunnel syndrome, restrictive or obstructive lung disease, and also scleroderma-like renal disease [54].

8.3 Histopathology

Scleromyxedema is characterized by diffuse deposits of mucin in the upper and middle part of the reticular dermis, increase in collagen deposition in the reticular dermis, and significant proliferation of irregularly distributed fibroblasts. Mucin may fill the walls of myocardial blood vessels as well as vessels of the kidney, the pancreas, adrenal glands, nerves, or lymph nodes [55].

8.4 Differential diagnosis

The primary differential diagnosis of scleromyxedema includes systemic sclerosis and scleredema. Other conditions in differential diagnosis with possible presence of mucin in the biopsy include nephrogenic systemic sclerosis. Differential diagnosis of leonine facies includes, for example, lepromatous changes, leishmaniasis, cutaneous lymphoma (T cell, rarely B cell), an actinic reticuloid as chronic actinic dermatitis, systemic amyloidosis, nodular mastocytosis, or sarcoidosis [53].

8.5 Treatment

Recommendations are still based on case reports and open-label small case series. Many chemotherapeutics, primarily melphalan, cyclophosphamide, methotrexate, or chlorambucil, have been tried, with no better results but with the risk of significant side effects. IVIg, alone or in combination with systemic medications such as thalidomide or systemic corticosteroids, may be administered as first-line therapy for cutaneous involvement and also systemic manifestations, including the dermatoneurological syndrome. Additional therapies include PUVA, UVA1, systemic retinoids, cyclosporine, electron beam radiation, plasmapheresis, and extracorporeal photochemotherapy with variable and unpredictable results [56].

9. Scleredema adultorum of Buschke

Scleredema is typically symmetrical diffuse induration and sclerosis of the upper part of the body especially of the trunk due to thickened dermis with mucin deposition and with relationship to diabetes mellitus.

9.1 Pathogenesis

Scleredema is a relatively unusual and rare disease that affects patients of all races. The typical form that is associated with diabetes mellitus is more prevalent in men, while other forms are seen more commonly in women. Irreversible glycosylation of collagen and resistance to degradation lead to an accumulation of collagen deposition. Furthermore, stimulation by insulin, microvascular changes and damage, and hypoxia during diabetes mellitus may increase the synthesis of collagen and mucin which result in a dermal deposition of collagen [57].

9.2 Clinical features

Scleredema adultorum may be divided into three clinical types of scleredema. The first type affects primarily children and middle-aged women. It is preceded by fever, malaise, and an infection (usually streptococcal) of the upper or lower respiratory tract. The localization of this type is the cervicofacial region with extension to the trunk and proximal upper limbs. The cervicofacial region typically affects the perioral localization with difficult opening of the mouth and hindered swallowing. This type usually resolves spontaneously. The second type shares the same clinical features as the first but with very slow manifestation and is more commonly associated with a monoclonal gammopathy [58].

The third type typically affects obese middle-aged men with insulin-dependent diabetes (scleredema diabeticorum). Sclerosis usually starts very slowly and the involvement is persistent. Affected skin is usually erythematous and indurated with typical localization of the posterior region of the neck and the back (**Figure 18**). The affected skin has peau d'orange appearance. In all three forms, systemic manifestations such as serositis, myositis, dysarthria, dysphagia, parotitis, and ocular and cardiac abnormalities may be present [57–59].

9.3 Histopathology

The main histopathological feature is the thickening of the reticular dermis, with atypical large collagen bundles. Mucin deposition is also present among separated collagen bundles. There is no increase in the number of fibroblasts, but the elastic fibers are significantly reduced in number. Mucin is also accumulated in the skeletal muscle and in the heart.

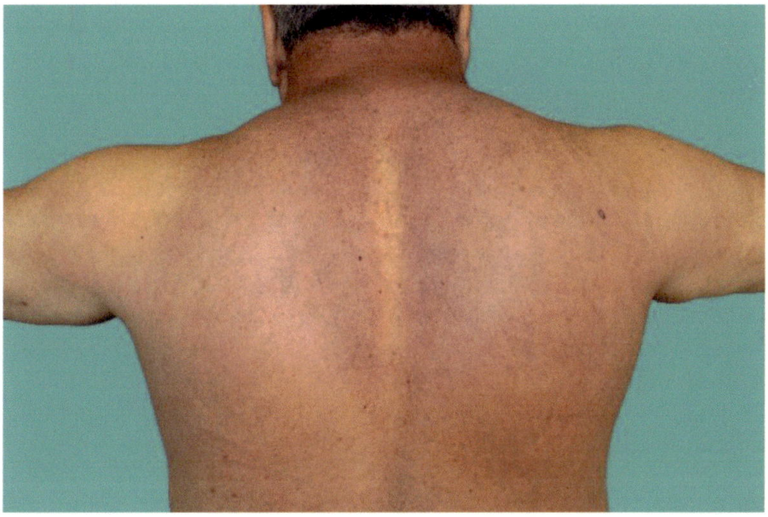

Figure 18.
Scleredema adultorum with typical localization of the posterior region of the neck and the back with affected erythematous and indurated skin.

9.4 Treatment

Scleredema which is associated with streptococcal infections is self-limited, thus no therapy is needed. Therapy of scleredema associated with diabetes or a monoclonal gammopathy is more difficult, and no specific treatment is available. Phototherapy as UVA1 or PUVA is the first-line therapy. Systemic and intralesional corticosteroids, intralesional hyaluronidase, antibiotics, methotrexate, cyclosporine, pulse therapy with cyclophosphamide plus oral corticosteroids, tamoxifen, and allopurinol have all been tried, with variable results [58, 59].

10. Endocrine disorders

Some endocrine disorders like diabetes mellitus and hypothyroidism can be accompanied with skin induration and sclerotic changes and may thus be a diagnostic problem for both systemic sclerosis and its localized forms. Endocrine disorders include sclerodactyly as "diabetic cheiroarthropathy" and myxedema in hypothyroidism.

10.1 Diabetic cheiroarthropathy

Diabetes mellitus is associated with a wide variety of rheumatologic manifestations which can significantly affect a patient's quality of life. One of these manifestations includes diabetic cheiroarthropathy which is associated with type I diabetes. Diabetic cheiroarthropathy affects typically the hands. It is postulated to result from increased glycosylation of collagen in the skin and is associated with retinopathy, nephropathy, and duration of the diabetes [60, 61].

10.1.1 Clinical features

Clinical features include thickened skin and limited joint mobility of the hands and fingers, leading to flexion contractures and an inability to approximate the palmar surfaces of the hands and fingers. Sometimes ischemic ulceration and calcinosis cutis can be present.

Treatment relies primarily on glycemic control and on nonsteroidal anti-inflammatory drugs and physical therapy with physiotherapy. With improved glycemic control, the symptoms and signs can be ameliorated and complete reversal is possible [61].

10.2 Mucinoses associated with thyroid dysfunction

Pretibial myxedema is characterized by cutaneous induration of the shins due to mucin deposition. It is often associated with hyperthyroidism most commonly due to Graves' disease. Localized myxedema with goiter, exophthalmos, and thyroid acropachy are typical signs of Graves' disease. Pretibial myxedema is found in 1–5% of patients with Graves' disease and in up to 25% of those with exophthalmos [62].

10.2.1 Localized myxedema

10.2.1.1 Clinical features

Localized myxedema presents as erythematous, yellowish or skin-colored waxy induration in a form of a nodulus or plaques. Typical localizations include ventral or

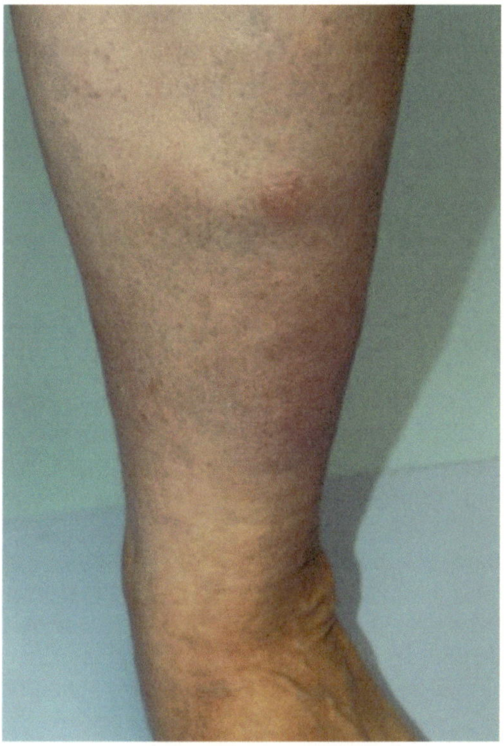

Figure 19.
Pretibial myxedema presents as erythematous waxy induration and nodulus on the ventral part of the shank.

anterolateral parts of the lower legs or the feet (**Figure 19**). In early phases localized myxedema can also present as a diffuse non-pitting edema of the shins or feet that evolves into lymphedema. Even more rarely, localized myxedema affects the face, shoulders, upper extremities, the lower abdomen, scars, or donor graft sites. Large plaques are often painful and pruritic. When present, hypertrichosis and hyperhidrosis are confined to the pretibial myxedematous skin [63, 64].

10.2.1.2 Treatment

First-line therapy such as topical corticosteroids or their application under occlusive dressings can be used. In some cases intralesional injection of corticosteroids can be effective. In a patient with lymphedema, medical treatments including IVIg, rituximab, plasmapheresis, and their combination with surgical treatment may have some benefit [63, 65].

10.2.2 Generalized myxedema

Generalized myxedema is a manifestation of hypothyroidism where mucin is deposited in the dermis, leading to waxiness of the skin. This condition is caused by a quantitative or functional deficiency of thyroxine. Impaired degradation of mucin and/or increased synthesis is suggested as the main cause.

10.2.2.1 Clinical features

The typical skin is pale, cool, waxy, and dry. Anhidrosis as an absence of sweating may lead to ichthyosis or eczema "craquelé." Hair and nails are dry and diffuse non-scaring alopecia is also common. A yellowish hyperkeratosis of the palms may be present. Sometimes purpura on the extremities and skin xanthomas may be observed [66].

10.2.2.2 Treatment

Early treatment of hypothyroidism is crucial for reduction or cessation of skin involvement and overall symptoms of the disease.

11. Amyloidosis

The cutaneous amyloidosis represents a heterogeneous group of conditions in which amyloid, as a fibrillar material that can result from the pathological degradation of various proteins, is deposited in the skin. In primary cutaneous amyloidosis, the deposits are derived from keratin (macular, lichen, biphasic) or immunoglobulin light chains (nodular) [67].

The specific cutaneous lesions of primary systemic amyloidosis are waxy, translucent, or purpuric papules, nodules, and plaques. Amyloid infiltration of the skin may produce thickening and stiffness. Typical localization may be on the limbs but sometimes also on the trunk. This is characteristic of AL amyloid, due to a plasma cell disorder in hematological malignancies. Primary systemic amyloidosis is due to a plasma cell dyscrasia, while secondary systemic amyloidosis arises from chronic inflammatory conditions such as rheumatoid arthritis or in the setting of chronic infections [67, 68].

Skin biopsy reveals accumulation of amyloid with characteristic staining (Congo red) properties under polarizing microscopic examination. Immunofixation of serum or urine is necessary for unambiguous identification of a monoclonal component [69].

Treatment of all forms of amyloidosis is challenging; although the primary cutaneous forms are not life-threatening, primary systemic amyloidosis can carry a poor prognosis for a patient [70].

12. Conclusion

Systemic sclerosis mimics include a variety of diseases that may resemble systemic connective tissue diseases such as SSc. Above all, the most common diseases are discussed in this chapter.

The basis of proper diagnosis and treatment is the interdisciplinary collaboration of rheumatology and dermatology with the possibility of biopsy tissue collection and histological verification of the disease.

A carefully performed clinical history and physical examination may distinguish these scleroderma mimic syndromes from systemic sclerosis (SSc, scleroderma) and from each other. The distribution and the quality/texture of skin involvement (in SSc typically: sclerodactyly, puffy fingers, ischemic defects/pitting scars/digital ulcers/gangrenes, telangiectasias, calcinosis), the presence of Raynaud's phenomenon (typically signs of a secondary Raynaud's phenomenon such as onset after the age of 40, asymmetry, thumb involvement, ischemic pain, history of symptoms <3 years, worsening attacks) or abnormal nail fold capillary microscopy (characteristic scleroderma patterns in SSc), the presence and type of associated systemic manifestations (typical organ involvement characteristic for SSc), and the association with particular concurrent diseases or specific laboratory parameters (SSc-specific autoantibodies such as anti-topoisomerase I, anti-centromere, anti-RNA-polymerase III) can be of substantial help in refining the diagnosis.

In some cases, a full-thickness skin biopsy is helpful to confirm the clinical suspicion. Effective therapies are available for some of these conditions, whereas others are more refractory. For this reason, a prompt diagnosis is important to guide treatment decisions wisely, to spare the patients from ineffective treatments, to facilitate appropriate diagnostic evaluations, and to allow for accurate determination of prognosis [71].

Acknowledgements

This chapter was supported by NV18-01-00161 A, MHCR 023728 and GAUK 312218.

Author details

Ondřej Kodet[1,2,3]* and Sabina Oreska[4]

1 Department of Dermatology and Venereology, First Faculty of Medicine, Charles University, Prague, Czech Republic

2 Institute of Anatomy, First Faculty of Medicine, Charles University, Prague, Czech Republic

3 BIOCEV, First Faculty of Medicine, Charles University, Vestec, Czech Republic

4 Institute of Rheumatology, Department of Rheumatology, First Faculty of Medicine, Charles University, Prague, Czech Republic

*Address all correspondence to: ondrej.kodet@vfn.cz

References

[1] Sehgal VN, Srivastava G, Aggarwal AK, Behl PN, Choudhary M, Bajaj P. Localized scleroderma/morphea. International Journal of Dermatology. 2002;**41**(8):467-475

[2] Gabrielli A, Avvedimento EV, Krieg T. Scleroderma. The New England Journal of Medicine. 2009;**360**(19):1989-2003

[3] Fett N, Werth VP. Update on morphea: Part I. Epidemiology, clinical presentation, and pathogenesis. Journal of the American Academy of Dermatology. 2011;**64**(2):217-228; quiz 29-30

[4] Peterson LS, Nelson AM, Su WP, Mason T, O'Fallon WM, Gabriel SE. The epidemiology of morphea (localized scleroderma) in Olmsted County 1960-1993. The Journal of Rheumatology. 1997;**24**(1):73-80

[5] Badea I, Taylor M, Rosenberg A, Foldvari M. Pathogenesis and therapeutic approaches for improved topical treatment in localized scleroderma and systemic sclerosis. Rheumatology (Oxford, England). 2009;**48**(3):213-221

[6] Yamane K, Ihn H, Kubo M, Yazawa N, Kikuchi K, Soma Y, et al. Increased serum levels of soluble vascular cell adhesion molecule 1 and E-selectin in patients with localized scleroderma. Journal of the American Academy of Dermatology. 2000;**42**(1 Pt 1):64-69

[7] Weibel L, Harper JI. Linear morphoea follows Blaschko's lines. The British Journal of Dermatology. 2008;**159**(1):175-181

[8] Niklander S, Marin C, Martinez R, Esguep A. Morphea "en coup de sabre": An unusual oral presentation. Journal of Clinical and Experimental Dentistry. 2017;**9**(2):e315-e3e8

[9] Tollefson MM, Witman PM. En coup de sabre morphea and Parry-Romberg syndrome: A retrospective review of 54 patients. Journal of the American Academy of Dermatology. 2007;**56**(2):257-263

[10] Sato T, Goto M, Takeo N, Hatano Y. Case of generalized morphea with the manifestation of diffuse systemic cutaneous sclerosis without sclerodactyly. The Journal of Dermatology. 2018;**45**(5):e100-e1e1

[11] Adamska U, Slinko A, Bialecka A, Mecinska-Jundzill K, Adamski P, Czajkowski R. Unilateral generalized morphea: A case report and literature review. Postępy dermatologii i alergologii. 2018;**35**(4):425-428

[12] Cantisani C, Miraglia E, Richetta AG, Mattozzi C, Calvieri S. Generalized morphea successfully treated with tacrolimus 0.1% ointment. Journal of Drugs in Dermatology. 2013;**12**(1):14-15

[13] Marzano AV, Menni S, Parodi A, Borghi A, Fuligni A, Fabbri P, et al. Localized scleroderma in adults and children. Clinical and laboratory investigations on 239 cases. European Journal of Dermatology. 2003;**13**(2):171-176

[14] Walker D, Susa JS, Currimbhoy S, Jacobe H. Histopathological changes in morphea and their clinical correlates: Results from the Morphea in Adults and Children Cohort V. Journal of the American Academy of Dermatology. 2017;**76**(6):1124-1130

[15] Zwischenberger BA, Jacobe HT. A systematic review of morphea treatments and therapeutic algorithm. Journal of the American Academy of Dermatology. 2011;**65**(5):925-941

[16] Stefanaki C, Stefanaki K, Kontochristopoulos G, Antoniou C, Stratigos A, Nicolaidou E, et al. Topical tacrolimus 0.1% ointment in the treatment of localized scleroderma. An open label clinical and histological study. The Journal of Dermatology. 2008;**35**(11):712-718

[17] Caca-Biljanovska NG, Vlckova-Laskoska MT, Dervendi DV, Pesic NP, Laskoski DS. Treatment of generalized morphea with oral 1,25-dihydroxyvitamin D3. Advances in Experimental Medicine and Biology. 1999;**455**:299-304

[18] Dytoc M, Wat H, Cheung-Lee M, Sawyer D, Ackerman T, Fiorillo L. Evaluation of the efficacy and safety of topical imiquimod 5% for plaque-type morphea: A multicenter, prospective, vehicle-controlled trial. Journal of Cutaneous Medicine and Surgery. 2015;**19**(2):132-139

[19] Kroft EB, Berkhof NJ, van de Kerkhof PC, Gerritsen RM, de Jong EM. Ultraviolet A phototherapy for sclerotic skin diseases: A systematic review. Journal of the American Academy of Dermatology. 2008;**59**(6):1017-1030

[20] Kreuter A, Gambichler T, Breuckmann F, Rotterdam S, Freitag M, Stuecker M, et al. Pulsed high-dose corticosteroids combined with low-dose methotrexate in severe localized scleroderma. Archives of Dermatology. 2005;**141**(7):847-852

[21] Ferreli C, Gasparini G, Parodi A, Cozzani E, Rongioletti F, Atzori L. Cutaneous manifestations of scleroderma and scleroderma-like disorders: A comprehensive review. Clinical Reviews in Allergy and Immunology. 2017;**53**(3):306-336

[22] Kirsner RS, Pardes JB, Eaglstein WH, Falanga V. The clinical spectrum of lipodermatosclerosis. Journal of the American Academy of Dermatology. 1993;**28**(4):623-627

[23] Stacey MC, Burnand KG, Bhogal BS, Black MM. Pericapillary fibrin deposits and skin hypoxia precede the changes of lipodermatosclerosis in limbs at increased risk of developing a venous ulcer. Cardiovascular Surgery. 2000;**8**(5):372-380

[24] Herouy Y, Kreis S, Mueller T, Duerk T, Martiny-Baron G, Reusch P, et al. Inhibition of angiogenesis in lipodermatosclerosis: Implication for venous ulcer formation. International Journal of Molecular Medicine. 2009;**24**(5):645-651

[25] Huang TM, Lee JY. Lipodermatosclerosis: A clinicopathologic study of 17 cases and differential diagnosis from erythema nodosum. Journal of Cutaneous Pathology. 2009;**36**(4):453-460

[26] Choonhakarn C, Chaowattanapanit S, Julanon N. Lipodermatosclerosis: A clinicopathologic correlation. International Journal of Dermatology. 2016;**55**(3):303-308

[27] Suehiro K, Morikage N, Harada T, Samura M, Nagase T, Mizoguchi T, et al. Compression therapy using bandages successfully manages acute or subacute lipodermatosclerosis. Annals of Vascular Diseases. 2019;**12**(1):77-79

[28] Bourrat E, Moraillon I, Vignon-Pennamen MD, Fraitag S, Cavelier-Balloy B, Cordoliani F, et al. Scleroderma-like patch on the thigh in infants after vitamin K injection at birth: Six observations. Annales de Dermatologie et de Vénéréologie. 1996;**123**(10):634-638

[29] Torrelo A, Suarez J, Colmenero I, Azorin D, Perera A, Zambrano A. Deep morphea after vaccination in two

young children. Pediatric Dermatology. 2006;**23**(5):484-487

[30] Slimani S, Ben Ammar A, Ladjouze-Rezig A. Connective tissue diseases after heavy exposure to silica: A report of nine cases in stonemasons. Clinical Rheumatology. 2010;**29**(5):531-533

[31] Zemtsov R, Zemtsov A. Porphyria cutanea tarda presenting as scleroderma. Cutis. 2010;**85**(4):203-205

[32] Partl R, Regitnig P, Tauber G, Potscher M, Bjelic-Radisic V, Kapp KS. Radiation-induced morphea-a rare but severe late effect of adjuvant breast irradiation: Case report and review of the literature. Strahlentherapie und Onkologie. 2018;**194**(11):1060-1065

[33] Perez-Lopez FR, Vieira-Baptista P. Lichen sclerosus in women: A review. Climacteric. 2017;**20**(4):339-347

[34] Dalziel K, Shaw S. Lichen sclerosus. BMJ. 2010;**340**:c731

[35] Kreuter A, Wischnewski J, Terras S, Altmeyer P, Stucker M, Gambichler T. Coexistence of lichen sclerosus and morphea: A retrospective analysis of 472 patients with localized scleroderma from a German tertiary referral center. Journal of the American Academy of Dermatology. 2012;**67**(6):1157-1162

[36] Oyama N, Chan I, Neill SM, Hamada T, South AP, Wessagowit V, et al. Autoantibodies to extracellular matrix protein 1 in lichen sclerosus. Lancet. 2003;**362**(9378):118-123

[37] Bunker CB. EDF lichen sclerosus guideline. Journal of the European Academy of Dermatology and Venereology. 2017;**31**(2):e97-ee8

[38] Wang JB, Yan H, Yang HY, Si JY, Jia LP, Li K, et al. Histopathological and ultrastructural changes of lichen sclerosus et atrophicus on the vulva. Chinese Medical Journal. 1991;**104**(10):868-871

[39] Staricco RG. Lichen striatus: A study of fifteen new cases with special emphasis on the histopathological changes and a review of the literature. A.M.A. Archives of Dermatology. 1959;**79**(3):311-324

[40] Singh L, Sengar M, Goyal S, Mansi M, Khurana N, Mohta A. Childhood phimosis secondary to lichen sclerosus: Is there a spatial pattern of histopathological changes? The American Journal of Dermatopathology. 2018;**40**(11):824-828

[41] Kai A, Lewis F. Long-term use of an ultrapotent topical steroid for the treatment of vulval lichen sclerosus is safe. Journal of Obstetrics and Gynaecology. 2016;**36**(2):276-277

[42] van der Avoort IA, Tiemes DE, van Rossum MM, van der Vleuten CJ, Massuger LF, de Hullu JA. Lichen sclerosus: Treatment and follow-up at the departments of gynaecology and dermatology. Journal of Lower Genital Tract Disease. 2010;**14**(2):118-123

[43] Lakhanpal S, Ginsburg WW, Michet CJ, Doyle JA, Moore SB. Eosinophilic fasciitis: Clinical spectrum and therapeutic response in 52 cases. Seminars in Arthritis and Rheumatism. 1988;**17**(4):221-231

[44] Onajin O, Wieland CN, Peters MS, Lohse CM, Lehman JS. Clinicopathologic and immunophenotypic features of eosinophilic fasciitis and morphea profunda: A comparative study of 27 cases. Journal of the American Academy of Dermatology. 2018;**78**(1):121-128

[45] Mazori DR, Femia AN, Vleugels RA. Eosinophilic fasciitis: An updated review on diagnosis and

treatment. Current Rheumatology Reports. 2017;**19**(12):74

[46] Smorodinsky E, Ansdell DS, Foster ZW, Mazhar SM, Cruite I, Wolfson T, et al. Risk of nephrogenic systemic fibrosis is low in patients with chronic liver disease exposed to gadolinium-based contrast agents. Journal of Magnetic Resonance Imaging. 2015;**41**(5):1259-1267

[47] Bruce R, Wentland AL, Haemel AK, Garrett RW, Sadowski DR, Djamali A, et al. Incidence of nephrogenic systemic fibrosis using gadobenate dimeglumine in 1423 patients with renal insufficiency compared with gadodiamide. Investigative Radiology. 2016;**51**(11):701-705

[48] Thomsen HS. Nephrogenic systemic fibrosis: A serious adverse reaction to gadolinium—1997-2006-2016. Part 1. Acta Radiologica. 2016;**57**(5):515-520

[49] Thomsen HS. Nephrogenic systemic fibrosis: A serious adverse reaction to gadolinium—1997-2006-2016. Part 2. Acta Radiologica. 2016;**57**(6):643-648

[50] Deng X, Chen F, Song Z, Yan H, You Y, Zhong B, et al. Four new cases of stiff skin syndrome with unusual presentations. Journal of the European Academy of Dermatology and Venereology. 2016;**30**(1):163-165

[51] Geng S, Lei X, Toyohara JP, Zhan P, Wang J, Tan S. Stiff skin syndrome. Journal of the European Academy of Dermatology and Venereology. 2006;**20**(6):729-732

[52] Guiducci S, Distler JH, Milia AF, Miniati I, Rogai V, Manetti M, et al. Stiff skin syndrome: Evidence for an inflammation-independent fibrosis? Rheumatology (Oxford, England). 2009;**48**(7):849-852

[53] Aoki M, Matsushita S, Kawai K, Kanekura T. Scleromyxedema clinically resembling to scleroderma. Indian Journal of Dermatology. 2016;**61**(1):127

[54] Nofal A, Amer H, Nofal E. Scleromyxedema without paraproteinemia. International Journal of Dermatology. 2016;**55**(7):e418-e419

[55] Rongioletti F, Rebora A. Cutaneous mucinoses: Microscopic criteria for diagnosis. The American Journal of Dermatopathology. 2001;**23**(3):257-267

[56] Saniee S, Davarnia G. Scleromyxedema without paraproteinemia: Treatment with thalidomide and prednisolone. Case Reports in Dermatology. 2016;**8**(3):327-332

[57] Meguerditchian C, Jacquet P, Beliard S, Benderitter T, Valero R, Carsuzza F, et al. Scleredema adultorum of Buschke: An under recognized skin complication of diabetes. Diabetes & Metabolism. 2006;**32**(5 Pt 1):481-484

[58] Kreuter A. Scleredema adultorum: Clinical presentation, diagnostic workup, differential diagnosis, treatment option. Hautarzt. 2018;**69**(11):908-915

[59] Cohn BA, Wheeler CE Jr, Briggaman RA. Scleredema adultorum of Buschke and diabetes mellitus. Archives of Dermatology. 1970;**101**(1):27-35

[60] Cherqaoui R, McKenzie S, Nunlee-Bland G. Diabetic cheiroarthropathy: A case report and review of the literature. Case Reports in Endocrinology. 2013;**2013**:257028

[61] Hider SL, Roy DK, Augustine T, Parrott N, Bruce IN. Resolution of diabetic cheiroarthropathy after pancreatic transplantation. Diabetes Care. 2004;**27**(9):2279-2280

[62] Fatourechi V. Thyroid dermopathy and acropachy. Best Practice &

Research. Clinical Endocrinology & Metabolism. 2012;**26**(4):553-565

[63] Brinster NK, Garrett AB, Kostopoulos TC. Localized myxedema of thyroid disease. Journal of the American Academy of Dermatology. 2013;**68**(6):e189-e190

[64] Katsambas A, Pantazi V, Giannakopoulou H, Potouridou I. Localized myxedema in Grave's disease confined to the toes. International Journal of Dermatology. 2000;**39**(12):953-954

[65] Dhaille F, Dadban A, Meziane L, Fessier C, Colta L, Lok C, et al. Elephantiasic pretibial myxoedema with upper-limb involvement, treated with low-dose intravenous immunoglobulins. Clinical and Experimental Dermatology. 2012;**37**(3):307-308

[66] Burman KD, McKinley-Grant L. Dermatologic aspects of thyroid disease. Clinics in Dermatology. 2006;**24**(4):247-255

[67] Palladini G, Merlini G. Systemic amyloidoses: What an internist should know. European Journal of Internal Medicine. 2013;**24**(8):729-739

[68] Schreml S, Szeimies RM, Vogt T, Landthaler M, Schroeder J, Babilas P. Cutaneous amyloidoses and systemic amyloidoses with cutaneous involvement. European Journal of Dermatology. 2010;**20**(2):152-160

[69] Nilsson KP, Ikenberg K, Aslund A, Fransson S, Konradsson P, Rocken C, et al. Structural typing of systemic amyloidoses by luminescent-conjugated polymer spectroscopy. The American Journal of Pathology. 2010;**176**(2):563-574

[70] Dember LM. Emerging treatment approaches for the systemic amyloidoses. Kidney International. 2005;**68**(3):1377-1390

[71] Varga J, Denton C, Wigley F, Allanore Y, Kuwana M. Scleroderma. 2nd ed. Cham: Springer International Publishing; 2017

Chapter 5

Sexual Dysfunction in Patients with Systemic Sclerosis

Barbora Heřmánková

Abstract

Systemic sclerosis (SSc) may affect all aspects of life including sexual function. Although sexual dysfunction is a neglected area of quality of life in patients with SSc, it turns out that it is an important issue for both men and women characterized by high prevalence. The etiology of sexual dysfunction in systemic sclerosis is multifactorial and includes factors associated with both physical and emotional (psychological) status. The most common physical problems in women are vaginal dryness, dyspareunia, and vaginal tightness. Erectile dysfunction is not only a frequent but also often underestimated clinical symptom in men with SSc. The incidence of erectile dysfunction in patients with SSc ranged from 12 to 81% in different studies. The main psychological factors that may affect sexuality are depression, fear, and changes in the appearance of the face and body that usually leads to impaired self-esteem. This chapter is a review about the impact of systemic sclerosis on sexual functioning.

Keywords: systemic sclerosis, sexual functioning, female sexual dysfunction, erectile dysfunction

1. Introduction

Systemic sclerosis is a chronic rheumatic autoimmune disease characterized by abnormal fibrotic processes, microvascular damage, and excessive deposition of collagen into connective tissues. The vascular alterations and immunological activation lead to progressive fibrosis of multiple organ systems including the skin, the gastrointestinal tract, kidneys, and the lungs. Disease-associated changes can have a negative impact on sexual functioning [1, 2]. Generally, sexuality in systemic sclerosis has been a neglected area so far, especially female sexual dysfunction. Impaired sexual functioning in women was probably less studied due to the complexity and multifactorial nature of female sexual response. A little bit more attention was paid to erectile dysfunction, where etiology is more pronounced even though women are affected by this disease more often [3–5]. The etiology of sexual dysfunctions in systemic sclerosis is not well known; the causes are multifactorial and are related to both the disease symptoms and the therapy. The most common physical problems associated with female sexual dysfunction include vaginal dryness, dyspareunia, vaginal tightness, Raynaud's phenomenon, fatigue, generalized pain, muscle weakness, joint contractures, heartburn, and dyspnea. Presence of depression, fear, changes in face and body appearance, and lack of self-esteem are the psychological aspects, which can play a key role in the pathogenesis of sexual dysfunction in systemic sclerosis patients [6]. The etiology of erectile dysfunction is a little bit more understood. It is considered to be a result of microangiopathic changes. Due to corporal fibrosis and myointimal proliferation, the blood flow in the penile arteries is reduced.

Several studies have suggested that sexual dysfunction is a widespread problem in both men and women with SSc. It is more prevalent than in general population and other chronic diseases [7]. The most common symptoms of female sexual dysfunction are vaginal tightness, dryness, and dyspareunia [7, 8]. More severe sexual dysfunction is usually associated with depression symptoms, aging, and functional impairment [2, 9, 10]. The prevalence of erectile dysfunction is about 80% [11–13]. In women, more than half of the SSc patients experience some sexual problems [7, 8]. The management of erectile dysfunction has been more studied compared to female sexual dysfunction treatment. However, the number of publications regarding the efficacy of erectile dysfunction treatment in SSc patients is still very limited and further research is needed. The treatment of female sexual dysfunction in SSc women has not been paid much attention so far. There are only general recommendations available.

2. Definition and classification of sexual dysfunction

In order to better understand why and how systemic sclerosis may affect sexual functioning, there is an overview of sexual response models, developed over the past few years, which led to the current diagnostic and classification criteria for sexual dysfunction. The first model of female sexual response was described by Masters and Johnson in 1966. They published that a normal female sexual response consists of four consecutive phases including desire, plateau phase, orgasm, and resolution. It was supposed that in both women and men, the sexual response is commenced by desire which is influenced by the activity of two brain centers—dopamine sensitive excitatory center and serotonin sensitive inhibitory center. These centers send a signal going through the descendent nervous system into the spinal cord from where the genital sexual reaction is triggered. The arousal phase is mediated by the parasympathetic nervous system, which leads to vascular and genital changes such as enlargement of the clitoris, dilatation of perivaginal arterioles, and lubrication and expansion of two-thirds of the vagina. The following level of excitement is referred to the plateau phase that lasts until the orgasm. The orgasm phase is accompanied by contractions of pelvic floor muscles, increased heart rate, respiratory rate, and blood pressure. After reaching orgasm, the body usually calms down and this phase is called the refractory or resolution phase (**Figure 1**) [14].

In 1979, this model was modified by Kaplan into a three-phase model, which consists of desire, arousal, and orgasm [15]. Based on this linear model, the diagnostic and classification system was developed. The World Health Organization International Classifications of Diseases-10 (ICD-10) and Diagnostic and Statistical Manual of Mental Disorders (DSM-IV) by the American Psychiatric Association were established. The ICD-10 focused on how physical factors influenced sexual response, whereas DSM-IV classification emphasized more emotional and psychological aspects of female sexual dysfunction. Because both approaches followed the linear model of sexual response, which was later criticized for not taking into consideration the complexity of female sexual response, the new classification was needed [16].

In 1998, the Sexual Function Health Council of the American Foundation for Urologic Disease (AFUD) convened an interdisciplinary congress, which was attended by 19 experts on female sexual dysfunction selected from five countries. The aim was to develop a consensual definition and classification based on the

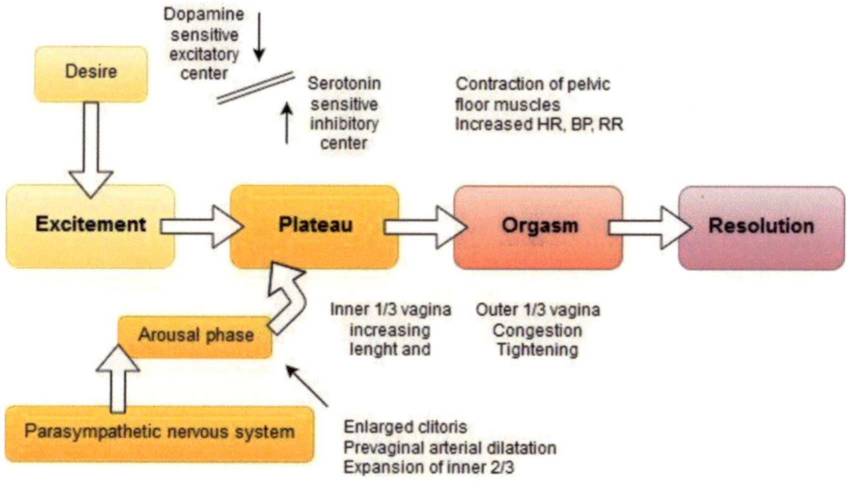

Figure 1.
The four-phase model of female sexual response cycle; BP = blood pressure, HR = heart rate, and RR = respiratory rate. Modified according to [14].

ICD-10 and DSM-IV. The new developed classification has been extended to include psychogenic and organic causes of desire, arousal, orgasm, and sexual pain disorders. An essential point of this classification is the personal distress criterion considering sexual complaint as a disorder only if it causes a subjective feeling of distress [17].

Further research has shown that the model of female sexual response is still incomplete and that many aspects affecting women's sexual function have been omitted. Studies reported that women often describe overlapping phases of sexual response in variable sequences. For instance, the unfounded assumption that desire always precedes arousal has been mistaken, and based on the women self-report and research data, it was proven that arousal and desire co-occur and reinforce each other. It was also found that motivation for sexual activity is much more complex than the mere presence of sexual desire defined as thinking or fantasizing about sex. Women in different surveys cited that increased desire for sexual activity may be caused by the emotional closeness of a partner or intimacy that increases female well-being and self-image, which may include the sense of feeling attractive, appreciated, loved, or desired. If enough appropriate sexual stimulation is provided, enough time and intimacy are available, the woman's enjoyment and excitement can be intensified. The type of stimulation, time needed, and interpersonal context are highly individual. Moreover, spontaneous desire can be affected by the menstrual cycle, which usually decreases with age and grows with a new relationship. These new findings have surpassed the original hypothesis that women's sexual response must always begin with sexual desire (thoughts and fantasies) and its absence is the result of a disorder. In addition, it was confirmed that, unlike men, there is no correlation between female subjective excitement and genital congestion. Subjective excitement could be influenced by interpersonal relationships, contextual factors, privacy, appropriateness, general emotional status, emotional relationships, biological factors, presence of depression, the influence of hormones (dopamine, testosterone), and others. In 2003, therefore, a revision of the current definition was done. The International Definitions Committee consisting of 13 experts from seven countries convened and proposed new definitions, which take into account new findings in the field of female sexual response [18–20].

Current definition was again revised in 2010 by the International Consensus of Sexual Medicine, where the movement away from the nonoverlapping linear model toward a more circular model depicting the variety of triggers of women's desire was accepted. It was emphasized that innate sexual fantasies and thoughts are not necessary for healthy sexual functioning and that desire is the result of sexual incentive that may be physically or subjectively perceived. Based on the previous findings, the arousal disorder was reclassified into subjective arousal disorder, genital arousal disorder, combined genital and subjective arousal disorder, and persistent genital arousal disorder. In May 2013, DSM-V was released, which also takes the focus away from the four-phase model, removed the sexual aversion disorder and merged vaginismus and dyspareunia into a new genito-pelvic pain/penetration disorder. It was finally noted that sexual dysfunction is a result of both psychological and biological and many other contributing factors [15, 21]. In 2015, the Fourth International Consultation on Sexual Medicine presented the new set of definitions of all forms of sexual dysfunction in women and men, which was based on ICD-10 and DSM-V (**Figure 2**) [22].

The newest changes in nomenclature of female sexual dysfunction came in May 2018, when the World Health Organization developed the eleventh revision of the International Classification of Diseases and Related Health Problems (ICD-11). The ICD-10 classification of sexual dysfunctions was separated to two main groups: "organic" and "nonorganic" conditions. The nonorganic sexual diseases were classified as mental and behavioral disorders and organic belonged to diseases of the genitourinary system chapter. However, since ICD-10 definition, lots of evidences have been accumulated regarding the causes of sexual dysfunction, which often involve a combination of physical and psychological factors. The ICD-10

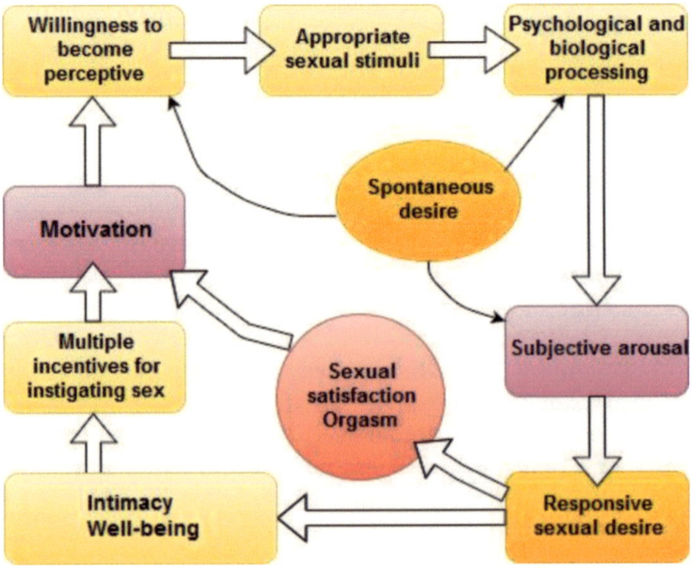

Figure 2.
Nonlinear model of female sexual response cycle. The initial stage of female sexual response is sexual neutrality, but with positive motivation (left). The reasons why a woman is willing to initiate or agree to sexual activity can be that she wants to feel loved, share physical pleasure or be emotionally closer to her partner, please her partner, or she wants to increase her own satisfaction. Stimuli for sexual activity are being processed in the woman's mind, influenced by biological and psychological factors, and result in subjective sexual arousal. If sexual stimuli last sufficiently long, sexual arousal and enjoyment will intensify, and it can trigger a desire for further sexual activity. It is important to note that desire appears at this point, not in the initial phase. When the stimulation continues and no negatives outcomes are involved, the process results in sexual satisfaction (with or without orgasm). Modified according to [23].

classification was therefore not consistent with clinical approaches in sexual health. ICD-11 diagnostic guidelines organize sexual dysfunctions into four main groups:

1. sexual desire and arousal dysfunctions;

2. orgasmic dysfunctions;

3. ejaculatory dysfunctions; and

4. other specified sexual dysfunctions.

Moreover, a separate grouping of sexual pain disorders has been established. Where possible, categories in this new classification of sexual dysfunctions apply to both men and women even though the differences in sexual response are known. On the other hand, the neural pathways and neurotransmitters mediating sexual response are the same for both men and women. Separate sexual dysfunction categories are provided where clinical manifestations differ [24].

The overview of current diagnostic criteria of sexual dysfunctions is presented below in **Table 1**. The present definition according the WHO ICD-11 is: "Sexual Dysfunctions are syndromes that comprise the various ways in which adult people may have difficulty experiencing personally satisfying, noncoercive sexual activities. Sexual response is a complex interaction of psychological, interpersonal, social, cultural and physiological processes and one or more of these factors may affect any stage of the sexual response. In order to be considered a sexual dysfunction, the dysfunction must: (1) occur frequently, although it may be absent on some occasions; (2) have been present for at least several months; and (3) be associated with clinically significant distress" [25].

ICD-11 (2018)	DSM-5 (2013)
Chapter: conditions related to sexual health	
Grouping: sexual dysfunctions	Grouping: sexual dysfunctions
Category: hypoactive sexual desire dysfunction	Category: female sexual interest/arousal disorder; male hypoactive sexual desire disorder
Category: sexual arousal dysfunction	Category: female sexual interest/arousal disorder
Category: orgasmic dysfunction	Category: female orgasmic disorder
Category: ejaculatory dysfunction	Category: erectile disorder
Subcategory: male early ejaculation	Category: premature (early) ejaculation
Subcategory: male delayed ejaculation	Category: delayed ejaculation
Category: other specified sexual dysfunction	Category: other specified sexual dysfunction
Category: unspecified sexual dysfunction	Category: unspecified sexual dysfunction
Grouping: sexual pain disorders	
Category: sexual pain-penetration disorder	Category: genito-pelvic pain/ penetration disorder

Table 1.
The eleventh revision of the International Classification of Diseases and Related Health Problems (ICD-11) and Diagnostic and Statistical Manual of Mental Disorders (DSM-5). Adapted from [25, 26].

3. Sexual functioning in women with systemic sclerosis

Persons with systemic sclerosis can experience a variety of symptoms that may affect all aspects of life, including sexual functions. The exact etiopathogenesis of sexual dysfunctions in systemic sclerosis is not well known; the causes are multifactorial and are related to both the disease symptoms and the therapy. Medical, pathophysiological, psychological, and social components may be involved in sexual dysfunction. Both physical and psychological problems arising from disease-related condition contribute to partnership difficulties, less active and less enjoyable sexual life [3, 27, 28].

The most common physical symptom is skin tightness. Due to skin tightness, the fingers becomes fixed in bent position, which could interfere with sexual foreplay, touch, and masturbation. If skin tightening causes the mouth to shrink, kissing or oral sex could become difficult. Sometimes the skin become stiffer around the vaginal introitus, which often leads to painful penetration, and changes in the vaginal mucosae causing lubrication disorder contribute to this [27, 29, 30]. Specifically, 56% of SSc female patients reported painful penetration during the intercourse [31]. The sexual difficulties such as vaginal tightness, dryness, and dyspareunia were reported by more than half of systemic sclerosis female patients [7, 8]. It was also published that vaginal tightness (71%), dyspareunia (56%), and ulceration (23%) were the most common symptoms of sexual dysfunction observed in 60 women with systemic sclerosis [31]. These genital tract abnormalities could be associated with a decrease in number and intensity of orgasm, which are also often observed in SSc individuals [32].

A majority of the systemic sclerosis patients experience Raynaud's phenomenon, which can affect not only fingers and toes but also tongue and nipples. This is another reason, why the cuddling, foreplay, and oral sex could become uncomfortable and unpleasant [27]. In addition, a lot of patients suffer from secondary Sjögren's syndrome characterized by drying of oral, nasal, ocular, and vaginal mucosae. The prevalence of Sjögren's syndrome in systemic sclerosis ranged in different studies from 20 to 69% depending on the criteria used and sample size. In Saad's study, 37% from 83 systemic sclerosis female patients reported Sjögren's syndrome, 56% of them had impaired sexual function, and vaginal dryness was the most presented symptom [29].

Another disease-related problem that impedes sexual activity is the affection of musculoskeletal system. The presence of joint contractures, stiffness, or pain leads to limited range of motion and it could restrict the ability to engage in sexual activities. Other aspects that reduced exercise capacity are muscle weakness and fatigue. It can be difficult to become sexually aroused when extremely tired. The consequence of skin thickening and other physical changes is the impaired body image, self-esteem, and sexuality. However, it has been also reported that body image dissatisfaction does not correlate with reduced sexual function [30]. In a different study, the major reasons for decreased sexual activity in married women with SSc were fatigue, altered body image, and pain [2]. Regarding psychological factors, depression is another often presented symptom that has been significantly associated with a sexual function disorder [8].

There are a few more causes that could lead to less active sexual life in SSc patients. For instance, in rare cases, the fibrotic process of visceral vessels leads to renal impairment that may have an impact on sexual desire and orgasm. It is usually the medication used to treat kidney problems rather than the problems themselves. Also, gastrointestinal problems such as heartburn or chronic diarrhea may disrupt sexual activities [7].

To sum up, existing studies of sexual function among women with SSc have concluded that sexual dysfunction is common in comparison to the general population. It was even showed a significantly greater decrease in orgasm and its intensity in SSc female patients compared to other systemic rheumatic diseases—rheumatoid arthritis and systemic lupus erythematosus [31]. What is more, Knafo et al. [4] published that the prevalence of sexual dysfunction is higher in SSc than in other chronic diseases such as breast cancer, gynecological cancer, or HIV positivity. On the other hand, Impens et al. [33] maintain that SSc women remain sexually active despite the psychological and physical difficulties caused by the disease. In this study, only 17% of women suffered from female sexual dysfunction primarily caused by systemic scleroderma. Other reasons for sexual inactivity were the absence of a partner (37%), personal choice (32%), and the health status of respondents' partners (20%).

4. Diagnostic approach of female sexual dysfunction

The first step in the diagnosis of female sexual dysfunction is a detailed personal, sexual, pharmacological, and psychosocial history. Where necessary, further examination by a psychiatrist, gynecologist, or physiotherapist is indicated. There are several objective methods assessing female sexual function, such as laboratory tests including hormonal profile or Doppler ultrasonography. However, laboratory tests in clinical practice are used only as auxiliary diagnostic methods. With duplex Doppler ultrasonography, it is possible to display a blood flow in cavernous tissue vessels, which is performed either under basal conditions or during sexual stimulations (vibrational or audiovisual) and objectified sexual arousal reactions. The most commonly used physiological method for evaluating sexual response is vaginal photoplethysmography, which investigates vascular reactivity during sexual arousal. It is based on the assessment of congestion of the vaginal mucosae. Other methods include electromyography, measurement of changes in vaginal pressure, and measurement of pH [34, 35].

Another widespread screening method is the questionnaire survey. Self-report questionnaires have a long history of use in psychological and sociological studies of sexual behavior. For example, Derogatis Sexual Function Inventory is a 245-item, multidimensional scale that evaluates a wide range of sexual behavior in 10 separate domains. Despite the very strong psychometric properties, this scale is not widely used in clinical trials due to its excessive length and complexity. Instead, several short evaluation scales have been developed [36, 37]. Currently, the female sexual function index (FSFI) is the "gold standard" in assessment of female sexual functioning [38]. FSFI is a widely used tool that has been validated for use across multiple populations including women of various age groups, in various health problems and sexual dysfunctions. It has been developed as a simple multidimensional self-assessment tool for assessing the key domains of female sexual function. The questionnaire consists of 19 items that evaluate sexual function over the last 4 weeks in six domains: sexual desire, sexual arousal, lubrication, orgasm, satisfaction, and pain [39]. Since the first validation study, it has been translated into more than 20 languages and validated in over 30 countries [40, 41].

It has to be noted that both objective methods and questionnaire screenings have their limitations. The main disadvantage of objective methods is the absence of an intimate condition that can play a key role in the female subjective arousal. Basson et al. published that intimacy and desire are essential to women's sexual activity. Raina et al. reported that intimacy leads to emotional arousal of a woman, followed by sexual desire and physical arousal that result in sexual satisfaction. These findings suggest that the presence of intimacy can be crucial in examining sexual arousal, and its absence can lead to a lack of emotional excitement and consequently to incomplete sexual responses [35, 42, 43]. On the contrary, the questionnaires are filled in private and evaluate women's real sexual experiences. Moreover, this method is not time-consuming and costly. However, as with any brief self-report scale of a complex psychophysiological construct, the questionnaire assessment has notable practical and theoretical limitations. Self-reported screening does not provide objective information but only patient's subjective perception.

In terms of FSFI, its drawback is the assessment of sexual activity in the past 4 weeks. Of course, there are number of reasons why women may be sexually inactive during a 4-week period and it does not necessarily imply significant sexual dysfunction. For example, the absence of sexual partner is a very common reason, why patients are not sexually active. Specifically, the FSFI questionnaire contains 15 questions, which could be answered "No sexual activity" or "Did not attempt intercourse." Both possible responses are scored as zero that could become problematic when lower scores indicate severer sexual dysfunction. In that case, the FSFI could produce biased results. Other inaccurate data may be the result of relatively vague terminology. A problematic issue seems to be to define and measure sexual desire and subjective sexual arousal. Studies suggest that women often have difficulty distinguishing desire and arousal in their sexual experience. Another drawback of the FSFI questionnaire is that questions in orgasm subscale are basically focused on the orgasmic function associated with penile-vaginal contact. In fact, the vagina is primarily a reproductive organ with little sensitivity, and clitoral stimulation is more important for female orgasm. Therefore, achieving orgasm should be judged more in conjunction with masturbation or oral sex than sexual intercourse [38, 44].

5. The use of the FSFI questionnaire in systemic sclerosis patients

The FSFI is also the most common questionnaire evaluating sexual function in women with systemic sclerosis. It has been used by an Italian team to evaluate the prevalence of sexual dysfunction in 46 women with SSc. The second purpose of this trial was to investigate the association with sociodemographic, physical, psychological, and disease-related variables. Compared to healthy controls, only the FSFI desire subscale score was significantly lower. The overall score did not substantially differ from healthy controls. The association with health status, functional ability, mouth affection, hand disability, and presence of depression was reported [10]. A very similar study has been conducted in the Netherlands. The FSFI was used to assess the sexual function of 69 SSc women aged 18–60 years. It was that the FSFI total score and the subscale scores for lubrication, orgasm, arousal, and pain were significantly lower in comparison with healthy population in the same age. Impaired sexual functioning and sexual distress were associated with marital distress and depressive symptoms [9]. Levis et al. first detected women with SSc who had engaged in sexual activities with their partner in the past 4 weeks, and then only sexually active patients completed a 9-item version of the FSFI. The aim of this Canadian cross-sectional multicenter study was to evaluate sociodemographic and clinical variables that distinguish sexually active from inactive patients and identify the source of pain during and after sexual activity in sexually active patients. The results showed that in total only 17% of 547 women were sexually active without sexual disorder [45]. The same group of scientists in different project used a shortened version of FSFI to compare sexual activity and impairment rates of women with systemic sclerosis to general population data. Among women with SSc, 296 of

730 (41%) were sexually active and 181 (61%) of sexually active patients reported sexual dysfunction. It means that only 115 of 730 (16%) patients engaged in sexual activities without impairment. It was also confirmed that SSc patients are significantly less likely to be sexually active and more likely to be sexually impaired than the general population of women [46]. Severe sexual dysfunction was also observed in married women with systemic sclerosis. About 8 out of 10 women achieved low scores in the FSFI questionnaire assessed, and all the subscales were affected in this study. The reasons why patients reported decrease in the frequency of intercourse since the onset of their disease and a diminished desire for a sexual relationship were fatigue, altered body image, and pain [2].

6. Treatment and recommendation for female sexual dysfunction

The management of female sexual dysfunction in the general population is based on the understanding of the basic physiology of female sexual response. Currently, several approaches of female sexual function treatment are available. It is known that some antidepressants can cause sexual dysfunction as a side effect. Antidepressants, such as SSRIs, are commonly associated with hypoactive sexual desire disorder (HSDD) and they have to be eliminated or dosed at lower levels. In women with major and disabling mood disorders, the adjustment of antidepressants requires a continuous collaboration with the prescribing psychiatrist, because dosage adjustments of antidepressants must be done very gradually [47]. Bupropion, buspirone, mirtazapine, vortioxetine, and vilazodone have been found to have lower rates of antidepressant-induced sexual dysfunction than other antidepressants, and they can be a suitable medication options for the treatment of depression [48–50].

Another option, primarily used in menopausal women, is hormonal therapy. Estrogen therapy may be used to increase clitoral sensitivity and libido and to reduce pain during and after sexual intercourse. In women with menopause-related sexual dysfunction that have estrogen treatment experience improved sexual desire, vaginal atrophy and vaginal dryness [49]. Transdermal estradiol has been found to be a preferred therapy for depleted estrogen. It is considered as the most effective therapy available for reducing vasomotor symptoms and associated menopausal symptoms with minimal adverse effects. Intravaginal estrogens combined with mechanical dilatations are also highly effective for treatment of vaginal atrophy [47]. Testosterone replacement therapy may also be considered to increase sexual desire and libido. Several high-quality sources documenting that transdermal testosterone is effective in restoring sexual desire are available [47]. Intramuscular testosterone combined with estradiol in postmenopausal women had a positive impact on sexual desire, arousal, and frequency of sexual fantasies compared with women without testosterone treatment [51].

Flibanserin is the first nonhormonal treatment for female sexual dysfunction to be approved by the Food and Drug Administration (FDA). The approval, in August 2015, occurred fully 18 years after the approval of sildenafil, the first treatment for erectile dysfunction. Flibanserin is a 5-HT 1A agonist and 5-HT 2A antagonist and is indicated for acquired hypo-active sexual desire disorder in premenopausal women. It is strongly recommended to avoid consumption of alcohol while using flibanserin treatment, because several serious adverse events were found: dizziness, loss of consciousness, hypotension, and circulatory collapse [49]. Another drug approved by the FDA is ospemifene, which is indicated in treatment of dyspareunia in postmenopausal women. It is a selective estrogen receptor modulator that can be prescribed when hormone replacement therapies fail. The daily dose of 60 mg of ospemifene has been found to be effective and tolerable for postmenopausal women with vaginal dryness and atrophy [52, 53]. To improve sexual functioning in domains of arousal, orgasm, and satisfaction, bupropion can be used, whose efficacy is based on the influence of dopamine and norepinephrine reuptake [54]. Although phosphodiesterase type 5 (PDE-5) inhibitors are mostly used in erectile dysfunction treatment, they can be used in women as well. Sildenafil has been found to significantly improve arousal, orgasm, and enjoyment in women without sexual dysfunction. In women with antidepressant-associated sexual dysfunction, sildenafil (in dose ranges of 50–100 mg) has also shown good efficacy [49].

Rehabilitation treatment can be useful in patients suffering from vaginism, dyspareunia, and anorgasmia due to pelvic muscle spasms. Adequate exercises can lead to normalization of muscle tension and relaxation [55]. Psychotherapy is recommended where the pathogenesis of sexual dysfunction has a psychological nature. Because recent studies have suggested that more severe sexual dysfunctions in patients with SSc are significantly associated with the presence of depression [2, 9, 10], the psychotherapy should be an integral part of the treatment of sexual dysfunction in SSc patients. In terms of sexual pain disorder, psychotherapy seems to be immediately helpful although objective research on the long-term efficacy of psychotherapy for sexual pain disorder is limited and difficult to evaluate [47].

There are some general recommendations for women with systemic sclerosis that may help to continue enjoying an active, fulfilling sexual life. If sexual activity is reduced due to pain, it can be alleviated by use of pain medication. The sexual activity can be scheduled for a time the pain will be at a minimum. A warm bath or shower before sexual activity often eases arthritic stiffness. The range of motion exercises before sex may help to reduce the stiffness. If the range of motion is limited and do not allow comfortable position, then it seems to be a good solution to experiment with sexual positions and try to find those that are the most suitable [3, 56]. If sclerosis has caused the mouth to shrink, physical therapist or occupational therapist can teach patients how to do the exercises to stretch the mouth. The regular stretching can improve the range of motion of the mouth and make kissing and oral sex more enjoyable. When fingers become fixed in a bent position, its possible to integrate stretching exercises as well and use the other part of hands (thumbs, wrists, or backs of the hands) to touch yourself or partner. An auxiliary material such as vibrators, creams, and lotions can also be used to enhance sexual activity. In order to avoid fatigue, patients with SSc may schedule their sexual activity for that part of the day when they still have enough energy, because becoming sexually aroused, when tired, is difficult. To prevent a Raynaud episode, it is necessary to keep entire body warm. It is possible to turn up the thermostat, leave some clothes on, or use extra blankets. When vaginal dryness and dyspareunia occur, the use of vaginal moisturizers on a regular basis along with lubricants as needed for sexual activity is the initial step in managing these symptoms. Women can choose from a number of commercially available lubricants that are either water based, mineral or plant oil based, or silicone based [47, 55]. Dilator therapy is an another option that can be useful in treatment of vaginal tightness. This method offers a nonsurgical approach to restore vaginal capacity and elasticity and alleviate sexual discomfort. If the penetration is still painful, there are alternative sexual activities like clitoral stimulation that can be sometimes more enjoyable than intercourse. If there is no interest in sex, still it is possible to stay physically close by holding or caressing one another [3, 56].

Several options for the treatment of female sexual dysfunction in normal population are available. The management of impaired sexuality in women with systemic sclerosis was less studied and the further research is strongly needed. What is essential and beneficial for the patients is the team-based model of care for management of sexual dysfunction including a medical provider, physical therapist, occupational therapist, psychotherapist, and sex therapist [57].

7. Sexual functioning in male with systemic sclerosis

Systemic sclerosis is an autoimmune connective tissue disorder characterized by following typical findings: endothelial changes, microangiopathic damages, and progressive fibrosis. These pathological processes may affect various organs including penile arteries leading to erectile dysfunction (ED). Male erectile dysfunction is defined as the consistent inability to reach and maintain an erection sufficient to permit satisfactory sexual performance. It is a widespread issue in men with systemic sclerosis. Sexual dysfunction in men has been given more attention than female sexual dysfunction, and the etiology is more obvious compared to women. Erectile dysfunction is a result of microangiopathic changes, when the blood flow is reduced in the small penile arteries due to corporal fibrosis and myointimal proliferation [5]. It was proven that damage of the penile cavernous arteries occurs in almost all SSc patients regardless of clinical symptoms. They are characterized by the presence of hyperechoic spots, suggesting fibrotic changes and low peak systolic velocities that are signs for vascular alterations [58].

The prevalence of erectile dysfunction in SSc patients ranged from 12 to 81% in different studies [28]. However, most studies agree that about 80% of SSc men are affected [11–13]. It was also found that ED is more prevalent in systemic sclerosis than other inflammatory rheumatic diseases. In a majority of men with systemic sclerosis, ED started to manifest after the onset of the disease. The mean duration from the onset of the first SSc symptom to erectile dysfunction was around 3 years [12]. Risk factors of erectile dysfunction such as smoking, hypertension, diabetes, and steroid use have been investigated. It was found that only self-reported history of nerve damage and diabetes are significant for predicting the likelihood of ED in systemic sclerosis. There are also risk factors that are presented in non-SSc men as well, like older age or alcohol consumption. The ED association with more severe diseases in terms of worse skin involvement, elevated pulmonary arterial pressures, presence of restrictive lung disease, and muscular and renal involvement in SSc patients was also confirmed [5, 12, 13, 59].

The most likely hypothesis of ED in SSc is a combination of vascular and fibrotic abnormalities. In men with SSc, decreased penile blood pressure, impaired peak systolic and diastolic blood flow in the penile arteries, and the presence of veno-occlusive dysfunction were found. Also, a decreased penile temperature and a slow recovery after cold exposure were reported. A duplex sonography was conducted to reveal the thickening of tunica albuginea and diffuse hyperechogenic spots within the corpora cavernosa. All these findings point to the microangiopathic cause of ED in male SSc patients. This is confirmed by the fact that no carotid artery thickening has been found in SSc, which would predict atherosclerotic macroangiopathy. From a histological point of view, the ED cause in SSc men is the presence of severe corporal fibrosis, increased collagen production by penile smooth muscle cells, and increased accumulation of extracellular matrix. Due to these changes, penile hypoxia arises, which can lead to overexpression of platelet-derived growth factor (PDGF), transforming growth factor (TGF)-β1 and TGF-β1 receptors in the corpora cavernosa, which are important profibrotic regulators of collagen synthesis and production of extracellular matrix. In addition, endothelin (ET-1) is also released by penile smooth muscle cells. Thus, penile hypoxia stimulates penile fibrosis. Therefore, it can be assumed that once ED in patients with SSc is manifested (due to disease), its next mechanisms are similar to those of non-SSc population. Other causes such as hormonal abnormalities or neurological causes have not been confirmed. No disturbances have been found in follicle-stimulating hormone, luteinizing hormone, serum testosterone, prolactin, estradiol, and thyroid hormones in SSc patients [5, 11, 59, 60].

8. Diagnostic approach of erectile dysfunction

The diagnosis of erectile dysfunction in SSc patients is not always easy. We are following the common steps starting with taking a detailed history. Then assessment with appropriate questionnaires and dynamic penile Duplex ultrasound is required. The ambiguity lies in the fact that penile vascular damage occurs in almost all SSc patients, regardless of clinical symptoms and the questionnaire results that often do not match with vascular findings. Thus, it is always better to carry out both investigations: the duplex ultrasound to document the degree of vascular involvement and self-administered questionnaire. The International Index of Erectile Function is the standardized and most widely used tool for evaluating erectile dysfunction. As mentioned above, penile temperature in SSc patients is lower than in healthy individuals. Since cutaneous temperature depends on cutaneous blood flow and thermal exchanges with deeper tissues, these findings could suggest the presence of functional alterations of both tissue properties and blood flow. Therefore, assessing changes in thermal properties and temperature control processes of the penis in SSc patients could provide a potential clue in diagnosis of erectile dysfunction. It has to be noted that with the progression of micro/macrovascular damage in the natural course of the disease, a concomitant penile fibrosis and veno-occlusive dysfunction occur and usually lead to difficult-to-treat ED. We should pay attention in cases where the reduced blood flow is observed, for example, on the hands (Raynaud's phenomenon), because it can suggest that the penile arterial flow will be also altered, and it may be a sign of initial stage of ED in SSc patients [61, 62].

9. Treatment and recommendation for erectile dysfunction

It is not a mistake to initiate ED treatment by eliminating general cardiovascular risk factors including lifestyle, psychological, or drug-related factors, but such treatment is often unsatisfactory. This step usually has beneficial effect on erectile function in the general population [63]. Phosphodiesterase-5 (PDE-5) inhibitors are recommended as a first-line option for pharmacotherapy. In non-SSc men, this group of drugs causes the relaxation of smooth muscle cells and temporarily increases arterial blood flow in the penis. However, to achieve an erection, sexual stimulation is required, because this class of drugs is not considered as an initiator of erection. Several types of PDE-5 inhibitors are currently available. The most commonly used are sildenafil (Viagra), tadalafil (Cialis), and vardenafil (Levitra). Except these, newer molecules of PDE-5 inhibitors can be used, for example, mirodenafil, udenafil, and avanafil. All types of PDE-5 inhibitors are effective and safe regarding the treatment of ED in the normal population. The differences are only in their half-lives, when, for instance, tadalafil is effective for up to 36 hours whereas the effectiveness of sildenafil is only 12 hours. The choice of a PDE5-I depends on the frequency of intercourse and the patient's personal experience [64, 65]. However, research on the efficacy of PDE-5 inhibitors is very limited in SSc patients [5]. Proietti et al. reported that once-daily tadalafil improved both erectile function and vascular measures of cavernous arteries in men with SSc-related erectile dysfunction. Also, an increase in frequency of morning erections and decrease in plasma ET1 levels were found. They suggest that daily tadalafil dose could play a potential role in preventing progression of penile fibrosis and erectile dysfunction in male SSc patients [58]. Furthermore, long-acting PDE-5 may lead to a decrease in the frequency and severity of Raynaud's phenomenon and the promotion of digital ulceration [66].

Patients who do not respond to PDE-5 inhibitors may be offered to try vacuum constriction devices. It was reported that patients who used the vacuum therapy system for a month to increase blood oxygenation in the corpora cavernosa and then employed the vacuum constriction device to maintain penile erection for sexual intercourse significantly improved their erectile function and sexual satisfaction [67]. However, there are no reports about the use of this system in patients with SSc.

Another option for the treatment of erectile dysfunction is prostaglandin analogues, which can be administered via intracavernous injections or intraurethral application. Alprostadil is a stable form of prostaglandin E1 that increases the concentration of cyclic adenosine monophosphate and decreases the intracellular calcium concentration, resulting in the relaxation of smooth muscle cells. Several studies reported the efficiency of alprostadil in the general population, but in terms of SSc patients, it was reported that a substantial percentage of SSc patients did not respond adequately to intracavernous prostaglandin E1 injections [68].

When pharmacotherapy fails and the patient wants a permanent solution, the surgical implantation of a penile prosthesis may be considered as the third-line option. Penile prosthesis improved erectile dysfunction in over 70% of men in the general population. Available prostheses are either malleable (semirigid) or inflatable (two or three pieces), but it should be considered that there are two main complications of penile prosthesis implantation—the mechanical failure and infection [5, 64, 65].

Most of the treatment options described above have not been verified in patients with systemic sclerosis yet. In spite of the fact that erectile dysfunction is common in men with systemic sclerosis, demographics, risk factors, and ED treatments have not been sufficiently investigated. Only a small case series has described unsatisfactory results with on-demand sildenafil (25–50 mg). The higher dose of sildenafil has not been investigated. Tadalafil has been slightly better evaluated in the treatment of SSc-related erectile dysfunction. The efficiency of 20 mg tadalafil on demand and 20 mg tadalafil in a fixed alternate day regimen has been compared. The results showed that flow-mediated dilatation and peak systolic velocities of cavernous arteries at penile duplex ultrasound improved significantly with the alternate day treatment; but no significant changes were observed after the on-demand tadalafil dosing. In addition, the alternate day regimen also reduced the plasma levels of ET-1 and vascular cell adhesion molecule as markers of endothelial function [68]. Therefore, long-term administration of tadalafil and its constant plasma level seems to have a positive effect on the treatment of ED in male SSc patients.

10. Conclusion

Sexual dysfunction is a common problem in both men and women with systemic sclerosis. Erectile dysfunction is the dominant issue in males, which seems to be tightly linked to vascular dysfunction. Sexual dysfunction in the female patient is not less prevalent, but it is considerably more complex and it has been less studied. Several diagnostic approaches have been established to assess sexual dysfunction. Also, there are some treatment options available, but most of them have not been sufficiently verified in patients with systemic sclerosis. Further research regarding sexual dysfunction in patients with systemic sclerosis is strongly needed.

Acknowledgements

This work was supported by grants AZV NV18-01-00161A, 16-33542A, 16-33574A, and institutional support of the Ministry of Health of the Czech Republic for the Institute of Rheumatology number: 023728 and GA UK 1578119.

Author details

Barbora Heřmánková
Faculty of Physical Education and Sport, Department of Physiotherapy, Charles University, Prague, Czech Republic

*Address all correspondence to: herman.barbora@gmail.com

References

[1] Heřmánková B. Sexual dysfunction in patients with systemic sclerosis. London: IntechOpen; 2019. DOI: 10.5772/intechopen.86219

[2] Frikha F, Masmoudi J, Saidi N, Bahloul Z. Sexual dysfunction in married women with systemic sclerosis. The Pan African Medical Journal. 2014;**17**:82

[3] Saad SC, Behrendt AE. Scleroderma and sexuality. The Journal of Sex Research. 1996;**33**(3):215-220

[4] Knafo R, Thombs BD, Jewett L, Hudson M, Wigley F, Haythornthwaite JA. (Not) talking about sex: A systematic comparison of sexual impairment in women with systemic sclerosis and other chronic disease samples. Rheumatology. 2009;**48**(10):1300-1303

[5] Jaeger VK, Walker UA. Erectile dysfunction in systemic sclerosis. Current Rheumatology Reports. 2016;**18**(8):49

[6] Carreira PE. A Female Scleroderma Patient with Sexual Dysfunction: Case Studies in Systemic Sclerosis. London: Springer; 2011. pp. 221-228

[7] Knafo R, Haythornthwaite JA, Heinberg L, Wigley FM, Thombs BD. The association of body image dissatisfaction and pain with reduced sexual function in women with systemic sclerosis. Rheumatology. 2011;**50**(6):1125-1130

[8] Sanchez K, Denys P, Giuliano F, Palazzo C, Bérezné A, Abid H, et al. Systemic sclerosis: Sexual dysfunction and lower urinary tract symptoms in 73 patients. La Presse Médicale. 2016;**45**(4):e79-e89

[9] Schouffoer AA, van der Marel J, Ter Kuile MM, Weijenborg PT, Voskuyl A, Vliet Vlieland CW, et al. Impaired sexual function in women with systemic sclerosis: A cross-sectional study. Arthritis and Rheumatism. 2009;**61**(11):1601-1608

[10] Maddali Bongi S, Del Rosso A, Mikhaylova S, Baccini M, Matucci Cerinic M. Sexual function in Italian women with systemic sclerosis is affected by disease-related and psychological concerns. The Journal of Rheumatology. 2013;**40**(10): 1697-1705

[11] Rosato E, Barbano B, Gigante A, Aversa A, Cianci R, Molinaro I, et al. Erectile dysfunction, endothelium dysfunction, and microvascular damage in patients with systemic sclerosis. The Journal of Sexual Medicine. 2013;**10**(5):1380-1388

[12] Hong P, Pope JE, Ouimet JM, Rullan E, Seibold JR. Erectile dysfunction associated with scleroderma: A case-control study of men with scleroderma and rheumatoid arthritis. The Journal of Rheumatology. 2004;**31**(3):508-513

[13] Foocharoen C, Tyndall A, Hachulla E, Rosato E, Allanore Y, Farge-Bancel D, et al. Erectile dysfunction is frequent in systemic sclerosis and associated with severe disease: A study of the EULAR Scleroderma trial and Research group. Arthritis Research and Therapy. 2012;**14**(1):R37

[14] Chen CH, Lin YC, Chiu LH, Chu YH, Ruan FF, Liu WM, et al. Female sexual dysfunction: Definition, classification, and debates. Taiwanese Journal of Obstetrics & Gynecology. 2013;**52**(1):3-7

[15] Latif EZ, Diamond MP. Arriving at the diagnosis of female sexual dysfunction. Fertility and Sterility. 2013;**100**(4):898-904

[16] Mimoun S, Wylie K. Female sexual dysfunctions: Definitions and classification. Maturitas. 2009;**63**(2):116-118

[17] Basson R, Berman J, Burnett A, Derogatis L, Ferguson D, Fourcroy J, et al. Report of the international consensus development conference on female sexual dysfunction: Definitions and classifications. The Journal of Urology. 2000;**163**(3):888-893

[18] Basson R, Leiblum S, Brotto L, Derogatis L, Fourcroy J, Fugl-Meyer K, et al. Revised definitions of women's sexual dysfunction. The Journal of Sexual Medicine. 2004;**1**(1):40-48

[19] Basson R, Leiblum S, Brotto L, Derogatis L, Fourcroy J, Fugl-Meyer K, et al. Definitions of women's sexual dysfunction reconsidered: Advocating expansion and revision. Journal of Psychosomatic Obstetrics and Gynaecology. 2003;**24**(4):221-229

[20] Basson R. Women's sexual function and dysfunction: current uncertainties, future directions. International Journal of Impotence Research. 2008;**20**(5):466-478

[21] Basson R, Wierman ME, van Lankveld J, Brotto L. Summary of the recommendations on sexual dysfunctions in women. The Journal of Sexual Medicine. 2010;**7**(1 Pt 2):314-326

[22] McCabe MP, Sharlip ID, Atalla E, Balon R, Fisher AD, Laumann E, et al. Definitions of sexual dysfunctions in women and men: A consensus statement from the fourth international consultation on sexual medicine 2015. The Journal of Sexual Medicine. 2016;**13**(2):135-143

[23] Basson R. Women's sexual dysfunction: Revised and expanded definitions. Canadian Medical Association Journal. 2005;**172**(10):1327-1333

[24] Reed GM, Drescher J, Krueger RB, Atalla E, Cochran SD, First MB, et al. Disorders related to sexuality and gender identity in the ICD-11: Revising the ICD-10 classification based on current scientific evidence, best clinical practices, and human rights considerations. World Psychiatry. 2016;**15**(3):205-221

[25] WHO. World Health Organization [Online]. 2018. Available from: https://icd.who.int/browse11/l-/en#/http://id.who.int/icd/entity/160690465 [Accessed: March 31, 2019]

[26] Association AP. Diagnostic and Statistical Manual of Mental Disorders (DSM-5®). American Psychiatric Pub; 2013

[27] Tristano AG. The impact of rheumatic diseases on sexual function. Rheumatology International. 2009;**29**(8):853-860

[28] Impens AJ, Seibold JR. Vascular alterations and sexual function in systemic sclerosis. International Journal of Rheumatology. 2010;**2010**:139020

[29] Saad SC, Pietrzykowski J, Lewis SS, Stepien AM, Latham VA, Messick S, et al. Vaginal lubrication in women with scleroderma and Sjogren's syndrome. Sexuality and Disability. 1999;**17**(2):103-113

[30] Bruni C, Raja J, Denton CP, Matucci-Cerinic M. The clinical relevance of sexual dysfunction in systemic sclerosis. Autoimmunity Reviews. 2015;**14**(12):1111-1115

[31] Bhadauria S, Moser DK, Clements PJ, Singh RR, Lachenbruch PA, Pitkin RM, et al. Genital tract abnormalities and female sexual function impairment in systemic sclerosis. American Journal of Obstetrics and Gynecology. 1995;**172**(2 Pt 1):580-587

[32] Sampaio-Barros PD, Samara AM, Marques Neto JF. Gynaecologic history in systemic sclerosis. Clinical Rheumatology. 2000;**19**(3):184-187

[33] Impens A, Rothman J, Schiopu E, Cole J, Dang J, Gendrano N, et al. Sexual activity and functioning in female scleroderma patients. Clinical and Experimental Rheumatology. 2009;**27**(3):S38

[34] Wylie K, Daines B, Jannini EA, Hallam-Jones R, Boul L, Wilson L, et al. Loss of sexual desire in the postmenopausal woman. The Journal of Sexual Medicine. 2007;**4**(2):395-405

[35] Basson R. Women's sexual desire—Disordered or misunderstood? Journal of Sex and Marital Therapy. 2002;**28**(1):17-28

[36] Rosen RC. Assessment of female sexual dysfunction: Review of validated methods. Fertility and Sterility. 2002;**77**(Suppl 4):S89-S93

[37] Brotto L, Atallah S, Johnson-Agbakwu C, Rosenbaum T, Abdo C, Byers ES, et al. Psychological and interpersonal dimensions of sexual function and dysfunction. The Journal of Sexual Medicine. 2016;**13**(4):538-571

[38] Stephenson KR, Toorabally N, Lyons L, Meston CM. Further validation of the female sexual function index: Specificity and associations with clinical interview data. Journal of Sex and Marital Therapy. 2016;**42**(5):448-461

[39] Wiegel M, Meston C, Rosen R. The female sexual function index (FSFI): Cross-validation and development of clinical cutoff scores. Journal of Sex and Marital Therapy. 2005;**31**(1):1-20

[40] Rosen RC, Revicki DA, Sand M. Commentary on "critical flaws in the FSFI and IIEF". The Journal of Sex Research. 2014;**51**(5):492-497

[41] Nowosielski K, Wróbel B, Sioma-Markowska U, Poręba R. Development and validation of the polish version of the female sexual function index in the polish population of females. The Journal of Sexual Medicine. 2013;**10**(2):386-395

[42] Raina R, Pahlajani G, Khan S, Gupta S, Agarwal A, Zippe CD. Female sexual dysfunction: Classification, pathophysiology, and management. Fertility and Sterility. 2007;**88**(5):1273-1284

[43] Basson R. Rethinking low sexual desire in women. BJOG: An International Journal of Obstetrics and Gynaecology. 2002;**109**(4):357-363

[44] Puppo V. Female sexual function index (FSFI) does not assess female sexual function. Acta Obstetricia et Gynecologica Scandinavica. 2012;**91**(6):759

[45] Levis B, Hudson M, Knafo R, Baron M, Nielson WR, Hill M, et al. Rates and correlates of sexual activity and impairment among women with systemic sclerosis. Arthritis Care and Research. 2012;**64**(3):340-350

[46] Levis B, Burri A, Hudson M, Baron M, Thombs BD, Canadian Scleroderma Research G. Sexual activity and impairment in women with systemic sclerosis compared to women from a general population sample. PLoS One. 2012;**7**(12):e52129

[47] Buster JE. Managing female sexual dysfunction. Fertility and Sterility. 2013;**100**(4):905-915

[48] Jacobsen PL, Mahableshwarkar AR, Palo WA, Chen Y, Dragheim M, Clayton AH. Treatment-emergent sexual dysfunction in randomized trials of vortioxetine for major depressive disorder or generalized anxiety disorder: A pooled analysis. CNS Spectrums. 2016;**21**(5):367-378

[49] Harsh V, Clayton AH. Sex differences in the treatment of sexual dysfunction. Current Psychiatry Reports. 2018;**20**(3):18

[50] Clayton AH, Pradko JF, Croft HA, Montano CB, Leadbetter RA, Bolden-Watson C, et al. Prevalence of sexual dysfunction among newer antidepressants. The Journal of Clinical Psychiatry. 2002;**63**(4):357-366

[51] Sherwin BB, Gelfand MM, Brender W. Androgen enhances sexual motivation in females: A prospective, crossover study of sex steroid administration in the surgical menopause. Psychosomatic Medicine. 1985;**47**(4):339-351

[52] Portman DJ, Bachmann GA, Simon JA, Ospemifene Study G. Ospemifene, a novel selective estrogen receptor modulator for treating dyspareunia associated with postmenopausal vulvar and vaginal atrophy. Menopause. 2013;**20**(6):623-630

[53] Portman D, Palacios S, Nappi RE, Mueck AO. Ospemifene, a non-oestrogen selective oestrogen receptor modulator for the treatment of vaginal dryness associated with postmenopausal vulvar and vaginal atrophy: A randomised, placebo-controlled, phase III trial. Maturitas. 2014;**78**(2):91-98

[54] Segraves RT, Clayton A, Croft H, Wolf A, Warnock J. Bupropion sustained release for the treatment of hypoactive sexual desire disorder in premenopausal women. Journal of Clinical Psychopharmacology. 2004;**24**(3):339-342

[55] Vegunta S, Kling JM, Faubion SS. Sexual health matters: Management of female sexual dysfunction. Journal of Women's Health. 2016;**25**(9):952-954

[56] Kocher A, Adler S, Spichiger E. Skin and mucosa care in systemic sclerosis–patients' and family caregivers' experiences and expectations of a specific education programme: A qualitative study. Musculoskeletal Care. 2013;**11**(3):168-178

[57] Rullo J, Faubion SS, Hartzell R, Goldstein S, Cohen D, Frohmader K, et al. Biopsychosocial management of female sexual dysfunction: A pilot study of patient perceptions from 2 multi-disciplinary clinics. Sexual Medicine. 2018;**6**(3):217-223

[58] Proietti M, Aversa A, Letizia C, Rossi C, Menghi G, Bruzziches R, et al. Erectile dysfunction in systemic sclerosis: Effects of longterm inhibition of phosphodiesterase type-5 on erectile function and plasma endothelin-1 levels. The Journal of Rheumatology. 2007;**34**(8):1712-1717

[59] Aversa A, Proietti M, Bruzziches R, Salsano F, Spera G. The penile vasculature in systemic sclerosis: A duplex ultrasound study. The Journal of Sexual Medicine. 2006;**3**(3):554-558

[60] Lally EV, Jimenez SA. Erectile failure in systemic sclerosis. The New England Journal of Medicine. 1990;**322**(19):1398-1399

[61] Merla A, Romani G, Tangherlini A, Di Romualdo S, Proiettii M, Rosato E, et al. Penile cutaneous temperature in systemic sclerosis: A thermal imaging study. International Journal of Immunopathology and Pharmacology. 2007;**20**(1):139-144

[62] Aversa A, Bruzziches R, Francomano D, Rosato E, Salsano F, Spera G. Penile involvement in systemic sclerosis: New diagnostic and therapeutic aspects. International Journal of Rheumatology. 2010;**2010**:706087

[63] Gupta BP, Murad MH, Clifton MM, Prokop L, Nehra A, Kopecky SL. The effect of lifestyle modification and cardiovascular risk factor

reduction on erectile dysfunction: A systematic review and meta-analysis. Archives of Internal Medicine. 2011;**171**(20):1797-1803

[64] Wespes E, Eardley I, Giuliano F, Hatzichristou D, Hatzimouraditis K. Guidelines on male sexual dysfunction: Erectile dysfunction and premature ejaculation. European Association of Urology. 2013;**2013**:1-54

[65] Hatzimouratidis K, Amar E, Eardley I, Giuliano F, Hatzichristou D, Montorsi F, et al. Guidelines on male sexual dysfunction: Erectile dysfunction and premature ejaculation. European Urology. 2010;**57**(5):804-814

[66] Shenoy PD, Kumar S, Jha LK, Choudhary SK, Singh U, Misra R, et al. Efficacy of tadalafil in secondary Raynaud's phenomenon resistant to vasodilator therapy: A double-blind randomized cross-over trial. Rheumatology. 2010;**49**(12):2420-2428

[67] Li P, Shen YJ, Liu TQ, Ma M, Zhang SJ, Wang YX, et al. Vacuum therapy for erectile dysfunction that fails to respond to PDE-5i: Report of 70 cases. Zhonghua nan ke xue = National Journal of Andrology. 2013;**19**(3):236-240

[68] Walker UA, Tyndall A, Ruszat R. Erectile dysfunction in systemic sclerosis. Annals of the Rheumatic Diseases. 2009;**68**(7):1083-1085

Chapter 6

Biopsychosocial Aspects in Management of Scleroderma Patients

Maja Špiritović

Abstract

Systemic sclerosis (SSc) is a rare, chronic connective tissue disease with characteristic fibrosis of the skin, musculoskeletal system, and internal organs. It is a heterogeneous and polymorphic disorder, in which fatigue, sleep disturbances, stiffness, and joint pain are among the most significant clinical symptoms. However, the presence of stiffening and thickening of the skin usually has a negative impact on the appearance of these patients, and the degree of self-dissatisfaction can fundamentally interfere with their personality. Self-consciousness and self-conception of the patient, accompanied by depression, can also be affected. Thus we cannot regard this disease and approach it only from a biomedical point of view and should not underestimate the approach to the psychosocial nature of the treatment. Biological, psychological, and social factors are interconnected, and imbalances in their complex interactions disrupt health and cause or worsen the disease. That is why it is necessary to create a so-called biopsychosocial comfort of an individual with SSc and to develop a number of activities in the sense of a complex treatment. This chapter focuses on the psychosomatic approach to health and illness and the development of the biopsychosocial model in medicine just as it should be used in patients with SSc.

Keywords: systemic sclerosis, biopsychosocial aspects, psychosocial aspects, psychosomatics, stress, non-pharmacological interventions

1. Introduction

Systemic sclerosis (SSc) is a disease in which fibrosis is one of the dominant pathological processes which affects the connective tissue, resulting in the involvement of the skin, musculoskeletal system, and internal organs. It is a very heterogeneous and polymorphic disease, and in each individual the course and extent of the involvement is different. Most of the characteristic visceral organ involvement, such as interstitial lung disease, pulmonary arterial hypertension, and cardiac and gastrointestinal involvement, has a significantly negative effect on physical fitness and condition. This decreased level of physical condition neither benefits from the thickening and rigidity of the skin nor from muscle and tendon contraction and stiffness of the joints accompanied by pain and an ever-worsening range of motion in the joints [1, 2]. Furthermore, the mind itself, as a result of such a physical condition, is not helping these individuals, and together with the body condition, they aggravate the quality of life of SSc patients in a mutually interacting fashion. In line with these principles, the healthcare professional's approach should be also targeted toward the body and mind (or soul) of the individuals with SSc, and only then can the treatment be successful.

2. Systemic sclerosis and its impact on the body and soul

Systemic sclerosis is a rare, chronic, and potentially lethal disease characterized by microvascular disorder, immune system activation, autoimmunity, and increased deposition of extracellular matrix components in the skin and internal organs [1–3]. To date, many mechanisms involved in the pathogenesis of SSc remain unclear, but there is increasing evidence suggesting that it is a complex pathological process, i.e., the interaction of the environment and genetic factors together with regulatory epigenetic mechanisms [1, 2, 4, 5]. Visceral organ involvement is responsible for increased mortality; however, in SSc patients, who are still alive, involvement of the lung, heart, skin, and musculoskeletal system poses a significant burden in terms of physical fitness and condition, as well as impairment of functional ability and quality of life [6, 7].

Non-pharmacological care for patients with SSc is becoming an increasingly important part of the interest of clinical research in SSc and is likely to reduce disability and improve the quality of life while contributing to the reduction of the burden of the disease. Overall, such care is predominantly focused on the musculoskeletal system and the skin [8]. Besides the physical component in the treatment of SSc patients, we must not forget the psychological (emotional) component (i.e., soul or mind) and the social components. These components are greatly and very often underestimated in the treatment, considerably subjective and different every other day, and therefore very demanding in research setting, but very useful in routine clinical praxis, if we, physicians or healthcare professionals, address them.

Every day, the organism is exposed to the effects of various stressors against which it is trying to resist and adapt to, such as viruses, bacteria, toxins (heavy metals), drugs, physical and psychological stress and the resulting lack of sleep, infection, responsibility, sadness, hunger, injury, the disease itself, etc. Each of us has a different ability to resist these stressors and thus to train the organism in the fight against them. However, if the burden of stress exceeds the effort of our organism, it leads to maladaptation, which results in negative consequences. It affects the psychological and physical state as well as the basic regulatory systems (hormonal, immune, and nervous) and leads to the onset of the disease or exacerbation of the disease itself. At the same time, we need some degree of stress to keep these regulatory mechanisms in place, for which we have to compensate with a certain degree of rest. Balance is the basis of good physical and mental health. Inability to rest to a right extent and form is one of the major factors in the development or worsening of a disease. Unfortunately, this is usually underestimated in clinical routine, where the treatment approach often deals only with the physical consequences of the disease. The patient is regarded as an object, not an entity that has its own way and means to help itself. And to better understand this principle, it is vital to explain two main concepts: movement and stress [9, 10].

2.1 Movement—the pillar of life in health and illness

Movement is a basic feature of life, and its disorder is a source of both somatic and psychological difficulties and significantly influences the motor behavior of a person regarding its physical, mental, and social aspects. The metabolic, digestive, excretory, hormonal, respiratory, and cardiac functions as well as reproductive organs also have a significant influence on movement behavior. However, the free movement itself is controlled by the nervous system [11]. Biocybernetics is a scientific discipline dealing with the description of these control processes. Its main purpose is to include different levels of living system information into a model enabling the understanding of the function of the living organism under physiological and pathological conditions, i.e., to split a human organism that is a complicated biological system into simpler parts that can be more easily described and interpreted so that the organism can be readily understood as a whole rather than an isolated organ or subsystem [12]. Thus, a two-way exchange and processing of information is being conducted between the brain and the executive motor and internal organs. This constitutes a psychophysiological correlate that cannot be divided. To put it simply, the brain sends information to the muscles as motor instructions, and the executive body sends sensory information back to the brain to assure that the instructions were executed. Nevertheless, the state of mind and the way of thinking also influence the course of the whole movement [11]. It is said that all living organisms have the ability to perceive and respond to changes in the external and internal environment by sensory and motor sensors. These changes are being continuously read by our brain, processed, integrated, and interconnected with our emotions and then, at the cortical level, allow us to become conscious of them and understand them. In addition to all this, the connecting nociceptive component is also important, e.g., painful inputs, which in most pathological conditions are associated with disorders of emotional and cognitive pain processing [9, 11]. Thus, every type of physical movement develops a specific type of reflective bodily consciousness that has a significant influence on how we feel our body and how we perceive the outside world. In other words, what we do with and to our bodies shapes the way we see and experience the world [13]. It is therefore important for contemporary science to perceive a person as a whole, i.e., as a functional unit, his soul (mind) and body, and in unity with the environment in which he lives. Furthermore, current science should limit the shortcomings in the sense of Descartes dualism, which is anchored in the history of medical knowledge and can be visible to this day [14, 15]. These two prevailing viewpoints in the treatment of an individual, body and soul, if they are apart from each other, are very limited. From the physical-mechanical point of view, it is a healing process that focuses on the physical structure of the organism and on the mechanics of movement at the site of the structure, and less attention is paid to other well-preserved structures. In this view, the mental influence on movement (caused by the developed disorder), considered to be a subjective accompaniment of movement, is neglected in the objective analysis of the mechanics of motion. On the other hand, from a psychological point of view, it is a treatment procedure focused on the evaluation of the movement function affecting the formation of the organ structure, as well as on the personality character and its influence on the movement behavior, which can cause motor failure [11]. Both viewpoints during treatment emphasize a certain component of movement and do not separately meet the condition of a comprehensive treatment approach. Such a holistic treatment approach and procedure should include both of these components. In the treatment of an individual, it should be very beneficial to both sides, to the patient and the healer, and eventually to the whole system and economy. We are no robots, thus we should neither divide "soma" from "psyche" nor "psyche" from "soma," neither in treatment nor in prevention.

2.2 Stress, our friend and foe

However, in order to maintain balance and life (movement, "psyche" and "soma"), it is important to adapt to various stressors acting on the living organism.

Despite the fact that ancient philosophers knew about stress and its effects, Hans Selye is considered to be the "father of stress." His well-known concept of general adaptive syndrome (GAS) refers to three levels of biological response to stress: (a) alarm reaction stage (fight or flight), (b) resistance stage (adaptive), and (c) exhaustion stage [16]. In his study of stress, Selye noted that patients with different illnesses had many of the same non-specific symptoms that were a common response to stressful stimuli and that long-term stress exposure led to adaptation disorders. Although the GAS hypothesis was subsequently shown to be incorrect, it has put stress on the map and also emphasized that stress has a major impact on the immune system and on the adrenal glands [17–19]. In addition, epidemiological studies dealing with stress confirm the association between fetal malnutrition or poor nutrition in early life and coronary heart disease and constant changes in glucose metabolism, resulting in the development of diseases of civilization such as type 2 diabetes and myocardial infarction [20, 21]. Similarly, advances in studying genes, which increase the vulnerability of individuals to stressful life events, have attracted considerable research interest. For example, polymorphism in the monoamine oxidase A (MAOA) promoter that reduces MAOA expression affects vulnerability to environmental influences. This biological process can be initiated by childhood abuse. Furthermore, polymorphism in the serotonin transport gene promoter can also make individuals more prone to stressful life events [22–24]. At the same time, neuroendocrinology research revealed that the autonomic nervous system and hypothalamic–pituitary-adrenocortical (HPA) system serve as means of the afferent and efferent limbs of the stress response in vertebrates and are also central for maintaining homeostasis and allostasis [19]. Nevertheless, there is no unambiguous definition of stress but different perspectives depending on the studied field and different conditions. Stress is based on two basic concepts: physiological, non-specific (based on general knowledge), and psychological, specific (based on the specifics of each individual). Thus we can say that stress is a universal concept that denotes any burden and any stress response leading to a violation of integrity, may it be supposed or true [25, 26]. According to Selye, stress is a non-specific (i.e., occurring stereotypically after a variety of stresses) physiological response of the organism to any requirement applied to the organism. He argued that stress is not identical to emotional excitement or nervous tension because stress can occur during anesthesia in humans or animals and may also occur in plants and bacteria that do not have the nervous system [27, 28]. Criticism of this definition has been subjected to an experimental test that has shown that each stressor has its own specific neurochemical signature. Since these stress indexes are limited to only two neurohumoral systems and since most stressors have at least some overlapping responses, it is not clear that this approach degrades Selye's definition. In addition, regardless of these limitations in the definition of Selye, cellular response to stress (in all living cells) is at molecular level represented by stress-induced synthesis of stress proteins or heat shock proteins (Hsps), of which molecular chaperones and proteases represent two well-characterized families. Many studies have shown that the response to heat shock is ubiquitous and highly conserved in all organisms from bacteria to plants and animals. It is a necessary defense mechanism for protecting cells (cytoprotection) from a wide range of stressors, including heat shock, alcohols, ischemia, energy metabolism inhibitors, heavy metals, oxidative stress, fever, or inflammation that, depending on amplitude and duration, can cause cell death by apoptosis or necrosis. Hsps also serve as modulation signals for immune and inflammatory responses and may play a role in the production of cytokines [19].

Selye also assumed that if the psychosocial aspect is as important to a human being as a biological aspect, its influence will have the same strength and consequences for the organism as biological factors. This has been later confirmed by new findings which demonstrate that psychological trauma has, in principle, analogous

DOI: http://dx.doi.org/10.5772/intechopen.86220

consequences to physical trauma. Thus the stress model has become an important tool of psychosomatic approach [29].

Nowadays, there is a lot of research and growing interest in stress research focusing on interactions between gene and environmental factors and the role of epigenetics and other mechanisms of gene control (e.g., RNA interference) in stress. This is also very important for research on rheumatic diseases, especially systemic sclerosis.

Systemic sclerosis is a disease, as we have indicated, where motion and locomotion are restricted, and the disease itself is a stressor. Let alone the disease itself could be triggered by a stressor in a genetically predisposed individual.

So now it can be clear that the presence of tissue fibrosis in patients with SSc may adversely affect the transmission of information from receptors in the skin, muscles, joints, intestines, blood vessels, etc. This can consequently adversely affect the perception of internal and external changes, i.e., transmission, processing, and integration of information from internal and external environments, and the subsequent response of the patient with SSc, which is usually accompanied by pain and emotionally narratively experienced by the patient on an individual basis. Such a physical state can have a negative impact not only on the motor behavior of the SSc patient but also on the state of mind and the way of thinking which, conversely, have an impact on the course of movement, self-perception, and the surrounding environment. Adaptation of the organism in such a diseased condition is then weakened by various stressors, and its perceptions and interpretations may be unfavorable. The extent of dissatisfaction with a visibly changing person, not only for the patient but also for other people in his surrounding, the reaction of which the patient perceives very negatively, basically interferes with the personality of the patient and interpersonal relationships, self-esteem, self-image, self-efficacy,

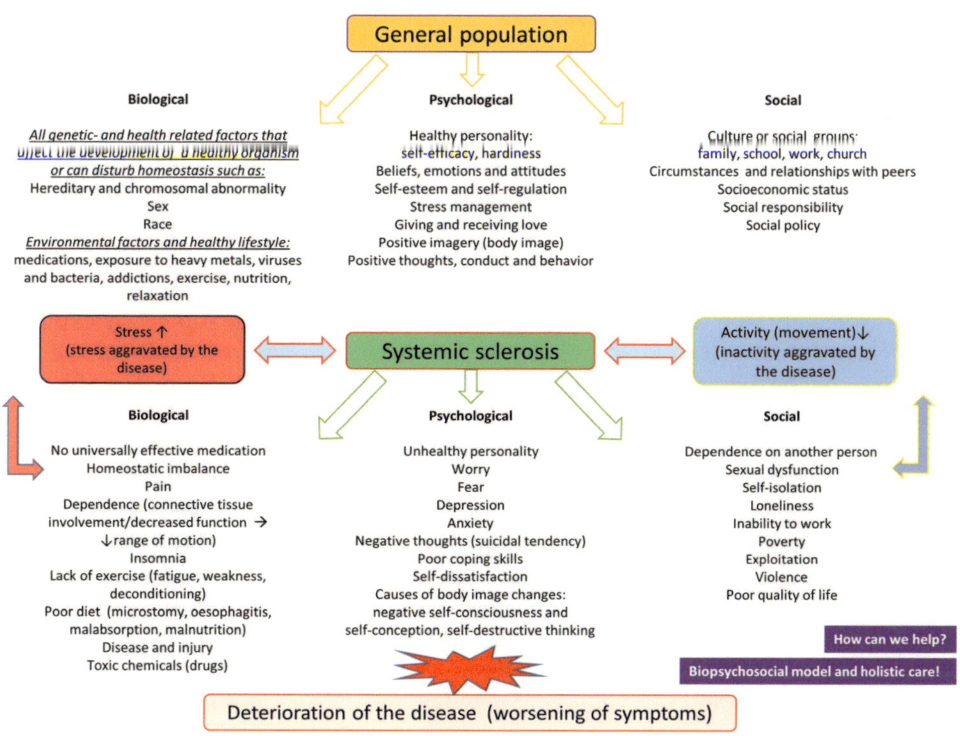

Figure 1.
Biopsychosocial interactions in general population and systemic sclerosis.

and socioeconomic position. To make the situation even more complicated, chronic fatigue; pain; disease-specific features, such as disease progression, severity, and related organ involvement; and subsequent reactive depression or anxiety greatly reduce the quality of life in SSc patients, as depicted in **Figure 1**.

2.3 Quality of life and its areas affecting the general condition of patients with SSc

As stated in the previous paragraph, there are a large number of symptoms accompanying SSc patients that affect the quality of life and are variably present on an individual basis, i.e., to a greater or smaller extent and with varying intensity and time course. All of them, however, have a negative impact on the entire biopsychosocial personality of the individual and are influenced by a number of physical, psychological, and sociocultural factors. A recent analysis of a large Canadian study found that the most frequently reported symptoms (out of 65 possible symptoms with moderate to severe impact on activities of daily living) by SSc patients (more than 450 in total) are fatigue (89–72%), Raynaud's phenomenon (86–72%), hand stiffness (81–59%), joint pain (81–64%), and sleep disorders (76–59%). Nevertheless, decreased hand function and joint and muscle pain have often been associated with a moderate to severe impact on daily activities. Fever, loss of appetite, weight loss, and reactive depression were also listed in the constitutional symptoms [30].

In a 2013 review of the studies on psychosocial aspects of SSc that were published in the literature following the publication of the Consensus Research Program in 2010, which reflected the limitations of available studies in this area, researchers used structured interviews to determine the prevalence of clinical mood disorders in SSc. It has been found that anxiety remains understudied, and distress may be a useful outcome to consider. Predictors of fatigue and sexual dysfunction in men and women with SSc have been identified. Furthermore, body image distress suggests the importance of changes in the facial skin and hands, and breathing problems and fatigue predicted workplace disability. The study also found the importance of multidisciplinary care for the quality of life related to health. The truth remains that after the publication of this Consensus Research Program in 2010, the research methodology in the SSc psychosocial area has improved; nevertheless, there is still no prospective study in this field. Interventions need to be developed and tested through randomized controlled trials with the power to detect clinically meaningful changes [31].

Evidence-based medicine (EBM) of factors and symptoms subjectively experienced is always very limited due to the complexity and reliability of its research. This is especially true for rare diseases such as SSc. However, the subjective experience of any disorder plays an important role in the subsequent projection of the symptoms of the disease. When searched for in scientific databases, published studies are often evaluating the quality of life, depression, fatigue, or pain in SSc patients. Yet, we all, physicians or healthcare professionals, if we have listened to patients and had that holistic approach, have certainly met many patients who complained not directly about depression or the quality of life but especially on pain, fatigue, sleep disturbances, a certain movement, functional limitations and inability, fear of the future, suicidal tendencies, shame in the circle of their friends, mouth opening problems, inability to work, sexual dysfunction, issues associated with pregnancy, etc. In addition, their psychosocial problems resulting from this disease could even somatize. We are well aware of several other issues that may play a role: anxiety that is not just a feeling but a whole range of chemical processes; presence of larval depression; variability of pain and its perception based on every individual experience; some forms of pain that are also mediated by the so-called

My fingers curl and I cannot properly close the fist, thus everything is falling out. I cannot open a bottle of water
At work, I do not want to shake the customer's hand. I could, but he would immediately notice and recognize that there is something wrong with my hands. That is why I am so ashamed of shaking people's hands
When someone squeezes my hand, then it hurts, and I make a painful grimace. Then he immediately knows that there is something wrong with my hands and I am ashamed
I cannot point at someone with the raised index finger, or point up the thumb to show someone thumbs up, or to make high five with somebody
I cannot scratch my back, but at least I can still wipe my behind
My ability to write with a pen has deteriorated, and my signature is constantly changing, which has been noticed by the staff in the bank
My face feels like a mask, and I feel that people around me realize that there is something wrong with my face. I can also tell the difference from the reactions of men: earlier, when they met me, they changed their behavior, straightened up, and tried to make a contact with me. Now they look like they do not see me at all
My mouth and tongue are becoming tightened, therefore it is more difficult for me to articulate, and sometimes I am being misunderstood. I cannot stick my tongue out at anyone
My eyelashes are falling out, thus I cannot apply paint to my lashes
To go out with friends for a dinner? I could, but I usually do not order any food because I know I would feel sick. I cannot have a wine because of heartburn. When I drink a beer, it comes back and I have a full mouth of bubbles. However, I can still do shots. Thus I mostly look like a fool, because I can only order still water, and everyone is asking me with sympathy, why I cannot eat. And then they feel sorry for me. Sometimes a piece of food falls out of my mouth
When on vacation, I have a problem eating at the hotel. Since my lungs are affected I cough every morning. When I go for a breakfast and start coughing, everyone looks at me and thinks I have tuberculosis or at least a contagious infection. Similarly, I get the same awkward feeling when traveling by a subway, bus or airplane. Usually I cannot eat much for dinner
I am not fit and able to climb a small hill
I cannot drink using a straw, whistle or lick my lips
My dentist is hysterical when he sees me. My teeth never used to decay easily, but now, even if I clean them very carefully, they do. I still have all four wisdom teeth and the dentist is afraid of repairing or extracting them since he cannot access them properly
When I had my picture taken for a new ID, I smiled a little. The clerk was making fun of me. I did not know why. Then he showed me the photo, if it was okay. I had a skewed smile. I told him that I always have a symmetrical smile, and that he should take a new photo. However, it was the same. When he did it once again, I eventually believed I looked this way
Because my esophagus is affected by scleroderma, I have to sleep in a semi-seated position, which is hard to organize in a hotel, which usually has a problem to get so many pillows for me. Thereafter, in the morning I walk hunched over from back pain
It annoys me when my friends, who have not seen me for a week, ask me, how I am doing. If my illness has improved. It bothers me when they feel sorry for me. I'd rather never have to meet anyone
I do not like to go anywhere, although prior to my illness, I could not stand it being without other people
My boyfriend left me because I could not satisfy him manually, orally, or vaginally. I'd rather die
Will my disease get worse when I deliver my baby?
I do not trust the doctors. I blame the contraception pills for triggering my illness
I have no friends anymore, because my physical condition is not what it used to be. They do not want to wait for me. When we should go outside for a walk, they rather say that they do not want to burden me, and that I should stay at home
I have two little children and I am afraid I will not be able to take care of them sooner or later. My husband left me
I am unable to work and am not financially secure. When I say I have a disease, no one wants to hire me

I have an affected esophagus and lungs, and digestive problems too. Other than that I do not look as a sick person. My biggest problem is fatigue, due to which I cannot normally function. Everyone thinks I am malingering. I have no support and I am in it on my own, and thinking about committing suicide
People are avoiding me
My breasts are gone
My skin is itching terribly and my face is full of small red spots
My skin color is changing, I look terrible
I cannot look in the mirror at myself anymore. It is not me.
There are only few specialists dealing with this disease and my doctor is very passive. I have to tell him what to prescribe
I live in countryside, and there is no physiotherapist available who could help me
I am not interested in any groups of patients with this disease. On one hand, they scare me, on the other hand, I feel alone. I want my normal life back. Will I ever have my old life back? Can I be healed?
I have researched this disease in the internet, where I found information that I would die within next 5 years. Is that true? If yes, I'd rather kill myself right now
On Facebook, I have read that stem cell transplantation can heal my disease. Is that true?
Do you think that alternative methods can help me? I have spent a lot of money already, and nothing has changed. What should I do? I do not want to die
I am unable to catch a bus or tram, since I cannot run, my lungs do not allow it. I am stiff, in pain and slow
What, do you think, would help you most in the treatment of your disease? Patients' answers: rest, option, freedom, peace, absence of introversion, contact with other people, experience, divorce, etc. (none of the patients said or thought about any potential new or existing drug!!!)

Table 1.
List of a few selected authentic sentences from the point of view of patients with SSc, which emphasize the need for a biopsychosocial model of the treatment of patients with SSc (from the author's own long-term experience with approximately 150 patients with SSc).

hidden central nervous system defects; chronic pain which always accompanies a change in behavior that often complicates and prolongs the course of the disease; some emotional or social problems which cannot be read well and are erroneously processed by a patient and then they are experienced in a physical form, etc. [9].

From my own experience, I particularly depict a few points of subjective experience in a few selected sentences articulated by the majority of more than 150 SSc patients during my 7-year practice that can be exhaustive for us healthcare professionals, but, on the other hand, they depict the everyday nightmare of patients with SSc (**Table 1**). This suggests that, aside from the EBM, SSc patients, if we listen to them, have psychological, emotional, social, and socioeconomic problems that should not be overlooked, because if they are not addressed, each of our treatment approach is wrong and we will not achieve the desired result. Thus, it is not enough just to direct the treatment in a biomedical manner, but it is necessary to aim, more extensively and as soon as possible, for the so-called biopsychosocial comfort of an individual. Therefore, interdisciplinary cooperation and the development of a number of activities in the area of complex rehabilitation are necessary in order to bring its significance to the attention of the wider medical community so that it becomes a necessary part of the treatment of patients with SSc in clinical practice.

3. Biopsychosocial model of the treatment of patients with SSc

Contemporary medicine should evolve to the ideal of a biopsychosocial (BPS) approach, i.e., psychosomatic treatment of patients, let alone its research. Because not just one, but all three factors (not separating emotions either), as we have suggested, precede some malfunction, experience, progression, and prognosis. In other words, "psyche" and "soma" form an integral and functional inseparable unit. Although in 1977 the World Health Organization (WHO) adopted a BPS model of illness involving biological, psychological, and social factors, which aims to extend the vision of a physician to psychosocial contexts, and to apply its practical use in everyday practice, there is still a long journey to a BPS model of treatment. It is due to the fact that one of the factors of increasing imbalance disfavoring psychosocial factors in ailing, besides its considerable complexity, can be the EBM methodology itself, which still favors biological factors in obtaining evidence of the correctness of the treatment [32]. The need for the BPS model of treatment was pointed out by Engel in the 1970s and 1980s [33, 34], who argued that the biomedical model of treatment does not take into account the psychosocial aspects of health and illness. He explained it by the fact that other factors (such as subjective experience of illness) that affect social, psychological, and cultural variables also interfere with biochemical responses and they need to be assessed in a view of their interaction with each other. Engel did not deny the importance of biomedical research in medicine, but criticized the too narrow (biomedical) focus of leading clinicians who see patients as objects and ignore the possibility that subjective patient experience is accessible to a scientific study. He promoted his ideas not only as a scientific proposal but also as a basic ideology that tried to reverse the dehumanization of medicine and the disarmament of patients. Furthermore, his research in psychosomatics has pointed to an integrative view, showing that fear, fury, neglect, and attachment have physiological and developmental effects on the whole organism [35]. According to him, the BPS model is a complex and systemic view of relationships that affect both health and illness both inside and outside the individual [36].

On the contrary, critics of the Engel's BPS model support Grinker's approach, which highlights biological factors that were otherwise ignored, especially in mental illnesses [36]. According to Monet and Lazarus, the BPS model is based on a stress theory that has a psychological and physiological level including the level of the environment [37]. And, according to Junne and Zipfe, there is a need for an interconnected biomedical and biopsychosocial approach and interdisciplinary cooperation [38]. Some authors think that the BPS model has helped patients to make better use of existing knowledge than the science itself in medicine [35]. Nevertheless, in 1977, the BPS model of illness was adopted by the WHO, which at the same time defined health as "a state of complete physical, mental and social well-being, and not merely the absence of disease or infirmity" [39].

Indeed, the definition is clearly indicated by the fact that if we want to heal or approach a healthy condition, an individual with SSc (or any other individual) must concentrate on maintaining a balance between these mutually affecting factors, which also jointly influence the onset, progression, and prognosis of the disease, its outcomes, and mortality of SSc patients. Biological factors in SSc comprise microvascular involvement of unknown etiology, immune activation, and progressive tissue fibrosis against which there is no universal effective drug available to date. In addition, more and more evidence points to a close link between environmental factors and the pathogenesis of SSc, i.e., the complete pathological process of interacting with the environment and genetic factors that corresponds to epigenetic mechanisms [3].

At the same time, fatigue, depression or anxiety, body image distress, pain, functional limitation, decreased quality of life, and disturbance of sleep patterns were noted among the main psychosocial factors influencing the adaptation to this chronic illness [31, 40–46]. Furthermore, from our own experience, in the history of patients, we can identify factors that precede the onset of the disease, namely, exposure to stressors and environmental factors, poor lifestyle or social support (family, society, and community), personality, emotional incompetence, etc. The question remains: Who is responsible for the treatment and resolution of these factors? The physician? Physiotherapist? Psychologist? Gynecologist? Sexologist? Occupational therapist? Social worker? Or some other healthcare professional? In the BPS model of treatment, the answer is clear—interdisciplinary cooperation which is very demanding but beneficial. And if there is no interdisciplinary cooperation, all of these factors (because these patients usually have them) fall into the care of one expert, who can experience a burnout or ignorance syndrome from exhaustion and great exertion and misunderstanding of all the components.

Unfortunately, the current concept of medicine addresses most of the patients (let alone patients with a rare and incurable disease like SSc) as an object from a biomedical point of view, assuming the linear relationship between the pathophysiology of the disease, its course, the patient's involvement, and disability, whose usual means of treatment are insufficiently effective. This is also the case if healing does not take place in a multidisciplinary team and the psychosocial factors affecting the ability of patients with SSc to face their disease are neglected and underestimated due to the idea that they belong to other professionals competent in this area. In addition, possible somatized psychosocial problems caused by this disease in SSc patients, who respect a physician who performs a social role for them which equals the position of God, strengthen this biomedical model most of the time. On the other hand, the psychosocial model assumes that the interdependence between the bio-, psycho-, and social variables is rather complex and therefore the SSc can be understood as a significant predictor of a mental condition. This is how we can say that such an integrated BPS model of SSc includes both the effects that contribute to the progression of the disease but also the influences involved in the disease behavior. However, none of the processes is linear but involves circular cycle and feedback with a repeating process over time [47–49].

From my own experience, I can point out that during the diagnosis process and subsequent treatment, the patient with SSc suffers from several stages of disease acceptance: from shock upon diagnosis, detection of its prognosis on inadequate web sites, anxiety states at the time of first physical symptoms and increased follow-up, inappropriate expectation of the results of further examinations to a depressive state of varying intensity. Another response is deciding whether to undergo treatment at all if there is no universal effective drug, and the drugs used to suppress the symptoms of the disease have many other undesirable and potentially toxic effects on the body. Consequently, some even experience maladaptation, refusal of treatment, and accompanying deep depression with suicidal thoughts. Nevertheless, the patient is constantly confronted with the reality of decreased life expectancy (70% of SSc patients survive for 10 years), the fear of pain, change in appearance, functional limitation, dependence on another person, loneliness, lack of social support, cessation of many activities, fear of treatment side effects, death, etc. Cognitive assessment of threats created by stressors and other possible sources has a central role in the effects of stressors on psychosocial and somatic outcomes.

In a 2014 study, where a personalized approach was used for modeling biopsychosocial features in relation to SSc-associated pain, the results indicated that psychosocial functioning is the basis for understanding the pain in this population, and physicians should apply the holistic approach and, if appropriate, recommend pain management in specialized centers [49].

And such a complex BPS model in SSc patients offers a comprehensive approach to diagnosis and treatment of its manifestations, including pain that mostly leads to suffering. However, suffering through somatization can also create pain, influenced by cognitive and emotional factors. This means that for a SSc patient, social and psychological impairment as a result of painful experience can be as difficult as somatic injury.

4. Conclusion

In conclusion, we can say that without the need to investigate EBM, an individual complex of biopsychosocial factors influences the onset, progression, treatment, and survival of SSc patients. In addition, besides the biological factors, the psychological and social factors play a significant role in negatively affecting the quality of life of patients with SSc and their interpersonal relationships, disruption and change of their personality and behavior, and coping with the illness. Since the illness and the consequences of treatment are reflected and manifested not only at the somatic level but also at psychological (emotional) and social levels, we should consider all these components in the treatment and approach in a multidisciplinary fashion. Since fatigue is one of the most prevalent symptoms which is adversely affecting the SSc patients, future research should investigate whether such a disease-associated depressive condition negatively promotes fatigue or whether effective pain management could reduce fatigue or explore other possible causes of fatigue and then find adequate strategies for its effective management. In any case, anyone involved in the treatment of SSc patients should have that twenty-first century holistic approach, take a proper medical history, and listen to patients' own opinions about their quality of health, which could help to spread the knowledge about psychosomatic correlations of the disease and adequate modification of the therapy for the patient. Nevertheless, proper education and awareness of the patient's illness is essential in managing the illness according to the best practice available.

Acknowledgements

This paper was supported by SVV for FTVS UK 2017-2019-260466, AZV 16-33574A, PRVOUK P38, and MHCR 00023728.

Author details

Maja Špiritović
Faculty of Physical Education and Sport, Department of Physiotherapy, Charles University, Prague, Czech Republic

*Address all correspondence to: spiritovic@revma.cz

References

[1] Denton CP, Khanna D. Systemic sclerosis. The Lancet. 2017;**390**(10103):1685-1699

[2] Allanore Y et al. Systemic sclerosis. Nature Reviews Disease Primers. 2015;**1**:15002

[3] Barsotti S et al. One year in review 2016: Systemic sclerosis. Clinical and Experimental Rheumatology. 2016;**34**(Suppl 100):3-13

[4] Manetti M, Matucci-Cerinic M. The new frontier in systemic sclerosis: From epigenetics to new treatments. In: Lu Q, Chang CH, Richardson B, editors. Epigenetics and Dermatology. 1st ed. Boston, Elsevier, Academic Press; 2015. pp. 487-504. ISBN 978-0-12-800957-4

[5] Broen JC, Radstake TR, Rossato M. The role of genetics and epigenetics in the pathogenesis of systemic sclerosis. Nature Reviews Rheumatology. 2014;**10**(11):671

[6] Mau W et al. Employment across chronic inflammatory rheumatic diseases and comparison with the general population. The Journal of Rheumatology. 2005;**32**(4):721-728

[7] Walker U et al. Clinical risk assessment of organ manifestations in systemic sclerosis: A report from the EULAR scleroderma trials and research group database. Annals of the Rheumatic Diseases. 2007;**66**(6):754-763

[8] Spiritovic M, Tomcik M. Non-pharmacological treatment in systemic sclerosis. In: Radic M, editor. Systemic Sclerosis. Split: InTech; 2017. pp. 85-111. ISBN 978-953-51-5045-9, ISBN 978-953-51-3547-0

[9] Červenková R, Kolář P. Labyrint Pohybu. Praha: Vyšehrad; 2018. p. 240. ISBN 9788074299957

[10] Kolář P. Rehabilitace v Klinické Praxi. Praha: Galén; 2009. p. 713. ISBN 9788072626571

[11] Véle F. Vyšetření Hybných Funkcí z Pohledu Neurofyziologie: Příručka Pro Terapeuty Pracující v Neurorehabilitaci. 1st ed. Praha: Triton; 2012. p. 224. ISBN 978-80-7387-608-1

[12] Bunc V. Biokybernetický Přístup k Hodnocení Reakce Organismu na Tělesné Zatížení. 1st ed. Praha: Výzkumný Ústav Tělovýchovný Univerzity Karlovy; 1990. p. 368. ISBN 807066214X

[13] Dincovici A. The appearance of the body: On body awareness and combat sports. In: Studia Phaenomenologica XII: Possibilities of Embodiment. Vol. 12. 2012. pp. 239-251

[14] Brown TM. Cartesian dualism and psychosomatics. Psychosomatics. 1989;**30**(3):322-331

[15] Damasio AR, Descartes' E. Emotion, reason and the human brain. Bulletin of the American Meteorological Society. 2002;**83**(5):742

[16] Miller FP, Vandome AF, McBrewster J. Fight-or-Flight Response: Walter Bradford Cannon, Theory, Animal, Threat Display, Sympathetic Nervous System, Priming, Combat, Stress (Biology), Vertebrate, Adrenaline Rush, Acute Stress Reaction. Alphascript Publishing; 2010. p. 68. ISBN 9786130608408

[17] Fink G. Stress: Definition and history. In: George F, editor. Stress Science: Neuroendocrinology. 1st ed. San Diego, CA: Academic Press; 2009. pp. 3-9. ISBN 9780123750662

[18] Hartl P. Stručný Psychologický Slovník. 1st ed. Praha: Portál; 2004. p. 252. ISBN 80-7178-803-1

[19] Fink G. Stress, definitions, mechanisms, and effects outlined: lessons from anxiety. In: George F, editor. Stress: Concepts, Cognition, Emotion, and Behavior. 1st ed. Amsterdam, Boston: Elsevier; 2016. pp. 3-11. ISBN 9780128009512

[20] Barker DJ. Fetal origins of coronary heart disease. British Medical Journal. 1995;**311**(6998):171

[21] Hales CN, Barker DJ. The thrifty phenotype hypothesis. British Medical Bulletin. 2001;**60**(1):5-20

[22] Caspi A et al. Role of genotype in the cycle of violence in maltreated children. Science. 2002;**297**(5582):851-854

[23] Caspi A et al. Influence of life stress on depression: Moderation by a polymorphism in the 5-HTT gene. Science. 2003;**301**(5631):386-389

[24] Caspi A, Moffitt TE. Gene–environment interactions in psychiatry: Joining forces with neuroscience. Nature Reviews Neuroscience. 2006;**7**(7):583

[25] Schreiber V. Lidský Stres. Praha: Academia; 1992. p. 80. ISBN 8020004580

[26] Bartůňková S. Stres a Jeho Mechanismy. 1st ed. Praha: Karolinum; 2010. pp. 137-ISBN 978-80-246-1874-6

[27] Selye H. A syndrome produced by diverse nocuous agents. Nature. 1936;**138**(3479):32

[28] Selye H. Confusion and controversy in the stress field. Journal of Human Stress. 1975;**1**(2):37-44

[29] Večeřová-Procházková A, Honzák R. Stres, eustres a distres. Interní Medicína Pro Praxi. 2008;**10**(4):188-192

[30] Bassel M et al. Frequency and impact of symptoms experienced by patients with systemic sclerosis: Results from a Canadian National Survey. Rheumatology. 2010;**50**(4):762-767

[31] Malcarne VL et al. Psychosocial aspects of systemic sclerosis. Current Opinion in Rheumatology. 2013;**25**(6):707-713

[32] Chvála V, Skorunka D. Bio-psycho-sociální přístup nabízí větší porozumění. Psychiatrische Praxis. 2017;**18**(1):42-46

[33] Engel GL. The need for a new medical model: A challenge for biomedicine. Psychodynamic Psychiatry. 2012;**40**(3):377-396

[34] George E, Engel L. The clinical application of the biopsychosocial model. American Journal of Psychiatry. 1980;**137**(5):535-544

[35] Borrell-Carrió F, Suchman AL, Epstein RM. The biopsychosocial model 25 years later: Principles, practice, and scientific inquiry. The Annals of Family Medicine. 2004;**2**(6):576-582

[36] Engel GL. The need for a new medical model: A challenge for biomedicine. Science. 1977;**196**(4286):129-136

[37] Monat A, Lazarus RS. Stress and Coping: An Anthology. 3rd ed. New York: Columbia University Press; 1991. p. 598. ISBN 0231074565

[38] Junne F, Zipfel S. Research prospects in BioPsychoSocial medicine: New year reflections on the "cross-boarder dialogue" paradigm. BioPsychoSocial Medicine. 2015;**9**(1):10

[39] World Health Organization. Preamble to the Constitution of the World Health Organization as adopted by the International Health Conference, New York; 19-22 June 1946; Signed on 22 July 1946 by the Representatives of 61 States (Official Records of the World

Health Organization, No. 2. p. 100) and Entered into Force on 7 April 1948; 1948. Available from: http://w\«v.who.int/abotit/3Ldefinition

[40] Mura G. Psychiatric symptoms and quality of life in systemic sclerosis. Clinical Practice and Epidemiology in Mental Health. 2012;**8**(1):30-35

[41] Malcarne VL et al. Medical signs and symptoms associated with disability, pain, and psychosocial adjustment in systemic sclerosis. The Journal of Rheumatology. 2007;**34**(2):359-367

[42] Jewett LR, Kwakkenbos L, Delisle VC, Levis B, Thombs BD. Psychosocial issues and care for patients with systemic sclerosis. In: Varga J, Denton CP, Wigley FM, Allanore Y, Kuwana M, editors. Scleroderma. Cham: Springer International Publishing; 2017. pp. 615-621. ISBN 978-3-319-31405-1

[43] Basta F et al. Fatigue in systemic sclerosis: A systematic review. Clinical and Experimental Rheumatology. 2018;**36**(113):150-160

[44] Thombs BD et al. Depression in patients with systemic sclerosis: A systematic review of the evidence. Arthritis Care & Research. 2007;**57**(6):1089-1097

[45] Hudson M et al. Health-related quality of life in systemic sclerosis: A systematic review. Arthritis Care & Research. 2009;**61**(8):1112-1120

[46] Thombs BD et al. Psychological health and well-being in systemic sclerosis: State of the science and consensus research agenda. Arthritis Care & Research. 2010;**62**(8):1181-1189

[47] Raudenská J. Biopsychosociální model léčby revmatoidní artritidy v algesiologii. Paliatívna Medicína a Liečba Bolesti. 2012;**5**(3):91-93

[48] Raudenská J. Biopsychosociální model onkologického onemocnění. Onkologie. 2011;**5**(4):244-246

[49] Merz EL et al. Biopsychosocial typologies of pain in a cohort of patients with systemic sclerosis. Arthritis Care & Research. 2014;**66**(4):567-574